WILD Habits

Unlock Your Mind, Improve Your Health,
and Release Your True Power

TARA MACKEY

SelectBooks, Inc.
New York

D1445920

This material has been written and published for educational purposes to enhance one's knowledge and ability to improve physical health and emotional and psychological well-being. The content of the book and recommendations given in the book are the sole expression and opinion of the author. The information given herein is not intended for the diagnosis of any medical condition, and the techniques presented here are not intended to be a substitute for an individual's prescribed medications or therapies. Apart from the author's personal experiences, no actual individual's experiences are recounted in the book, but are composites based on experiences of multiple individuals. All cases and examples of people's experiences and claims of good health results from ingesting supplement products are the sole opinion of the author, and the publisher does not recommend or endorse any supplement products from any source. When making a choice to engage in an exercise or diet regime, individuals should always consult their personal physician and other medical professionals they work with.

This edition published by SelectBooks, Inc.
For information address SelectBooks, Inc., New York, New York.

First Edition

ISBN 978-1-59079-445-6

Library of Congress Cataloging-in-Publication Data

Names: Mackey, Tara, 1986- author.
Title: Wild habits : unlock your mind, improve your health, and release your
   true power / Tara Mackey.
Description: First edition. | New York : SelectBooks, [2018] | Includes
index.
Identifiers: LCCN 2017037061 | ISBN 9781590794456 (paperback book : alk.
paper)
Subjects: LCSH: Mackey, Tara, 1986- | Naturopathy. | Health. | Alternative
medicine. | Mind and body.
Classification: LCC RZ440 .M3337 2018 | DDC 615.5/35--dc23 LC record
available at https://lccn.loc.gov/2017037061

Book design by Janice Benight

Manufactured in the United States of America
10 9 8 7 6 5 4 3 2 1

For Dad
You still guide my life in every way.

*"Have self-control, master all of your senses,
act with wisdom, conquer life and find freedom."*

—PARAMAHANSA YOGANANDA
Journey to Self Realization

CONTENTS

Introduction

Drugs are in my DNA. I was born on hard drugs, and I spent my first two weeks in the NICU—newborn rehab. My mother was an addict, and my father was out of the picture, so I encountered some tough emotional situations as a child. Because of this, I found myself on many different prescription medications as a young adult. Unfortunately I believed many of the labels assigned to me and allowed my diagnoses to truly become my identity. And even though deep down I knew something wasn't right, that this dizzying medley of disorders did not sound like the true me that I knew, that the prescription drugs all made me feel worse instead of better, I felt completely powerless to change or improve.

If you've picked up this book, you may be familiar with this feeling. The feeling of being completely powerless is one of the most relatable experiences in the world. It's both terribly lonely and uncomfortable and yet incredibly universal and tangible. We've all been there.

I know that by the end of our journey together, if you apply just *some* of the methods and knowledge that you'll gain throughout this book, you can conquer that powerless feeling completely. By practicing the simple new rituals that you'll learn about in these pages, you can transform your life.

You can take control of your health and win the war against your own mind—if only you knew how! Many people who read my bestselling first book, *Cured by Nature*, had the same follow-up question. *That's inspiring that you overcame all of your odds,* they said. *That's incredible that you recognized what was hurting you. That's amazing that you took your health into your own hands and got your life back.* But, they wanted to know: *How?* How, exactly, did I stop the addictions that were killing me? How have I resisted turning back to harmful habits for seven years? How did I build the willpower? How did I replace my bad habits with good ones? How have I built successful businesses, and how do I live a healthy, vibrant life, making an income doing what I love?

This book is the How.

It's not written in chronological order of what I went through (although that story will be told). This book is written in the order that will best illustrate the properties that make the method work. It's written in a way that will make it easier for you to implement these techniques into your life. I've picked topics that make the most difference along the way: your past, your energy, your nutrition, movement, wealth, meditation practice, personal relationships, health, and success. I'll take you through my personal story, plus the stories of many of the folks that WILD habits have saved and changed for the better. I know that with these stories to learn from, you'll be more capable of surrendering to your highest good.

I've written this book for you in three easily digestible parts. While we explore some powerful and, at times, complicated concepts, I have done my best to keep things in a conversational tone. I know firsthand that taking your health or your life back can be intimidating, so I've tried to make your WILD habits and the WILD Method as easy to understand and implement as possible.

Part 1 introduces you to the WILD Method and explains what your WILD habits are. This part is essential to building a framework for the rest of the book—and the rest of your life! Once you can identify your harmful habits versus your WILD habits, we'll discuss ways that you can recognize and change your life and build a plan to be successful that is completely unique to you.

Part II explores the power of your mind and teaches you techniques for mind-body connection that will keep you on track for a more abundant, joyful existence. These techniques are explored technically, philosophically, and scientifically, so you'll understand not just what to do, but how to do it successfully and for the long term.

Part III provides you with WILD strategies to remain disciplined, natural remedies that can replace the most common drugs on the market today, as well as tried-and-true tips and tricks for long-term prosperity. These strategies will make your harmful habits easier to recognize and enable you to incorporate your new habits effortlessly into your life. The remedies we'll delve into have worked effectively to cure many of the ailments I used to treat with medication, and they've worked miracles for countless others, going as far back as history can take us. I implore you to dig into them with an open mind and heart.

Once you have the strategies of Part III coupled with the identification methods from Part I and the mind-strengthening techniques from Part II, you'll possess incredible tools to heal a variety of issues, from past trauma to chronic pain, anxiety, and depression; from toxic friendships and addiction to coping with a devastating loss. We'll explore how you can find relief through the abundance of medicine that nature has to offer you, to treat many ailments we face on a day-to-day basis. You'll discover the most important ways to ensure long-term success in your relationships, family dynamic, health, business, and so much more. You'll finish this book with tools you never knew you had and a powerful arsenal in your pocket to combat any circumstances life may throw your way.

I woke up one day and realized that I was no longer truly living—and that moment changed my life. I was finally able to see past the diagnoses, labels, and prescriptions, trust my own instincts, and use the power of my mind to help heal my body naturally. I learned how to replace my unhealthy habits with healing, WILD habits that have brought abundant joy to my life. I don't want anyone to live a life of misery the way I did for far too long. My greatest hope is that this method can help you to experience true health and happiness—now and for the rest of your life.

The Danger of Labels

I was prime real estate for diagnoses and medications. Orphans, children, minorities, and women have all been used as human experiments for new drugs since the beginning of recorded medical history. Not only did I feel like a human experiment, it seemed I literally was one. Additional illnesses, labels, and medications dripped into my life every few months after my first diagnosis. By my late teens in college, I was taking eight different pharmaceuticals a day.

I received my first label in 2001 and knew almost no one who had the same diagnosis: bipolar disorder. On record today, more than five million people in the United States are currently diagnosed as bipolar. It is the second most common mental illness diagnosed in the United States, and Mayo Clinic now says there are more than three million cases of bipolar diagnosed *per year*. However, it appears from research studies that this may be an over diagnosis, because primary care physicians—not psychiatrists—are now prescribing bipolar medications to treat symptoms without in-depth psychiatric examinations. There are serious risks involved when placing a patient on a psychiatric drug that may not be right for them and that may also have major ramifications when they try to wean themselves off of it.

For a long time, I gave in to the idea that I was powerless. I was convinced that I was powerless to my past, powerless to my circumstances, and most of all, powerless to my own mind. I willingly defined myself by my past experiences, by my health, by my labels, by my family history, and by my genetics. I even identified myself *by my illnesses*. "Hi, I'm Tara and I'm bipolar!" Though I may not have ever actually *said* it, that was the vibe I exuded at every opportunity. I didn't have to say it. I was living it. I indoctrinated my illnesses into my identity. With a diagnosis and a long list of presumptions about "how I should act" under my belt, I powerfully attracted illness and toxicity into my life at every turn by constantly focusing on it.

Every time I left the house, my purse rattled with pills. Birth control, painkillers, mood stabilizers, benzos for anxiety, muscle relaxers, and nerve blockers were for daily use. Every other orange bottle was to be opened and used "as needed."

Despite this daily concoction, which was undoubtedly meant to *help* me, I was trying very hard day in and day out not to admit that *somehow* I was still hurting and I was still struggling. Big time.

In my case, everything that had happened previously in my life piled up to a daily weightiness. Pills were all I knew. Pharmaceutical medication was all I believed in and the only answer that I had ever learned to tackle my feelings of helplessness. Yes, I had been to many therapy sessions. I had learned my fair share of coping mechanisms growing up: talking it out, drawing, writing, and listening to music.

I also frequently watched an hour of *Oprah* after school throughout my childhood. As Ms. Winfrey interviewed (and helped beyond belief) those with similar and much less fortunate circumstances than I found myself in, I felt a lot less alone. I learned how others dealt with the most devastating things that could happen to them. I saw the light come back into people's eyes. I watched people get their lives back. I was always so inspired after that hour was up. I looked up to Oprah as a mentor and an angel, put on this earth specifically to help those in need. I wondered if I'd ever be one of those people—the kind of person who finally receives help and then is fortune enough to find themselves with a platform that allows them to help others.

Besides Oprah, my uncle gifted me cassettes and books by larger-than-life coach Tony Robbins (now more famous for his net worth and Netflix documentary than his infomercials, which dominated the late-night TV circuit in the 80s and 90s). Tony became my go-to mentor and a sane voice in the dark, confusing world I lived in as a kid. His booming voice echoed throughout my whole childhood. I played his tapes and CDs over and over and over again until I had memorized them. I read and reread his books, which had more yellow highlighted parts than not. I pictured a day where the circumstances Tony spoke about would manifest. I dreamed about having control of my life, having a family I was proud of, and accomplishing goals that were dear to my heart. This hope helped me more than I may ever be able to express.

And yet at age twenty-one I was on ten different prescription drugs, including a popular sleeping pill, Ambien. Ambien would often assign my brain to sleep while my body was still up and active. I had a handful of near-fatal accidents and made a lot of unfortunate personal choices during blackouts on this drug, with no recollection of the events. Soon enough, I had a dozen labels and a dozen pills a day to go with them—all with my name on them: Dilaudid, fentanyl patches, Valium, Oxycodone, Ativan, Klonopin, Lyrica, Seroquel, Celebrex, Flexeril, and more. I told doctors what was wrong with me and they responded with "take another pill." While I did not take all of these drugs at once, most days I was swallowing at least eleven pills throughout the day.

I was a genetics major in college, and I found that I knew more about drug classification than most other premed students, not because I was blessed, but because I had been on almost every kind of medication that you can name.

As my circumstances grew darker and my mind became cloudier, the mechanisms I had to cope got lost in the fog. There were years I never thought to turn to these coping mechanisms at all. I shunned self-help and nonfiction books during college in favor of hard science and psychology textbooks, hoping to explain my own neurosis. I ignored the copies of *Awaken the Giant Within* by Robbins, which I had carried with me from bookshelf to bookshelf for almost twenty years, in favor of researching the side effects of my latest Rx drug. Truthfully, the more pills I piled on, the less I was inspired to turn to these amazing mentors or indulge in good habits in the first place. The small glimmers of comfort that were so essential to me as a child were no match for the power of eleven years of constant drugs combined with living in an unforgiving emotional landscape.

By the age of twenty-four I'd already been on this roller coaster for almost half of my life. I was familiar with the entire process from start to finish. I knew every twist and turn and stomach drop of the ride.

Real Effects

Getting a label from a doctor always led to taking another pill, which eventually led to a conspicuous side effect like dizziness, trouble concentrating, migraines, dehydration, disorientation, depression, pain, or anxiety. This would send me back to that doctor, which led to an appointment with another doctor to address my side effects. This ultimately led to more prescriptions, more trips to the pharmacy, more bottles of pills rattling in my purse, and more effects from the new drugs.

Days were bleeding into nights. Months were coasting unnoticed into years, with more stress added on and less accomplishments checked off. My to-do list was daunting, ever-growing, and nearly always included a doctor's appointment. Every bone ached.

As time went on, my vision became desaturated and dull. My organs were shutting down, and my liver was overworked. Kidney infections were popping up every few weeks. My school work, creativity, and relationships all suffered. With every gulp of pharmaceutical medication I said a small, desperate, silent prayer: *Help me.*

Every new side effect I experienced soon led to taking another pill to treat myself for another new ailment. It was endless, and no matter what kind of doctor I saw, what sort of clinic I went to, or what my symptoms were, I left with a prescription and wound up at home with a bottle of pills and a Bible-sized encyclopedia of side effects and directions.

Unfortunately for me, it felt like nothing worked. You see, a doctor may tell you that the "side effect" of your medication is weight gain or seizures or blackouts or suicidal tendencies, but your body doesn't know the difference between "side effects" and effects. "Side effects" are just effects. To our bodies, they are all very potent effects. I call them *real effects.*

I had been blasting my body with real effects from medication for eleven years, and I was only in my early twenties. I would take each medication and then deal with the real effects: seeing the correct doctors, taking antibiotics or anti-inflammatories, and bargaining with my organs not to shut down. I wound up in the hospital plenty of times for dehydration, anxiety attacks, sepsis, and organ infections—all prolonged effects of pharmaceutical drug use. During this time in my life, I never even thought to ask my doctors to wean me off these drugs completely. Anytime I even hinted at a decreased dosage or a med switch, my doctors scrunched their noses and justified my plethora of pills by saying I "needed them." They called wanting to come off my medication "a symptom of my illness." I had an illness and I just had to deal with that. Medication was presented as the best—and only—option that I had. I was told that without medication I simply wouldn't have a life, build relation-ships, do well in school, or succeed, despite the glaring fact that I had done all of those things perfectly well before starting meds. It was only after I started medication that I developed any personal or learning problems. Before that, it was mostly my tumultuous environment that had been the culprit in my unhappiness. After meds, it was mostly myself.

Once you've been typecast as a child with problems, and car-ried a mental diagnosis throughout your life without "fighting" it, it becomes harder and harder to fight against that diagnosis as a grown or growing adult. Not only have you labeled your thoughts and feelings under your diagnosis but also you have literally fed into your symptoms since receiving your label. Chances are, you believe you are sick. You believe you are whatever they tell you that you are. They're professionals, after all.

It's hard not to believe the professionals. I came to learn how difficult it truly is. Before deciding to come off my medication com-pletely, I had consulted with my doctors in New York. Each time, I was met with one of two responses:

1. A doctor will agree to adjust your dosage.

2. A doctor will agree to put you on a different medication.

For them, there was no in-between.

Discovering the Universal Tools to Wellness

My scientific background taught me a whole lot about the human body, but virtually nothing about health. In all my days analyzing human anatomy, chatting with patients, squinting through microscopes, and calculating challenging equations, I learned absolutely *zilch* about what my body truly needed to function properly.

I scored jobs at prestigious hospitals and laboratories in New York City by passing their assessment and aptitude tests with flying colors. By my early twenties, I had more certifications in my field of biology than I could easily recall, and I had worked in nearly every medical study of interest—from fertility to maxillofacial surgery. I had learned a lot about how these medical settings worked, but I can say honestly that I had gained absolutely no knowledge about how to care for myself or truly invest in another's health during my studies, internships, and scientific career.

I never learned, for instance, how to access my energy level. I was never taught how to stop when I had overexerted myself. I had no way of knowing how to *listen* to my body. I wasn't instructed on what to eat to fuel myself or how to be kind when another person might need it. I wasn't even encouraged to be kind to myself when I might need it. I don't think I ever heard the word "self-care." Not one time.

Although I learned the names, purposes, and applications of many pharmaceutical drugs in my schooling, I mastered virtually nothing about how these drugs truly worked for the ailments they were invented to treat. I wondered a lot about what was truly *in* Lamictal, Flexeril, and Dilaudid, and how they did what they did. What the heck had I been ingesting almost every single day for the last ten years of my life? Lamictal isn't on the periodic table of elements—so what exactly was in this pill and *why*, for instance, was it blue?

I was committed to discovering as much as I could about what I had been putting in my body and how it might have affected my health. In 2011, when I had finally buckled down and made the decision to examine my own personal wellness regimen, I wondered if there were any natural, healthy alternatives to treat myself for pain, mood fluctuations, sadness, and anything else I had taken pills for in the past. I had a lot of questions, and I was about to be blown away when I learned their answers.

When I finally took the leap and decided to break up with my meds—every single one of them, immediately, and for good—I was soon bedridden from withdrawal. But I was determined to learn. With this determination, my life came into alignment in ways that had eluded me for years. Books on natural healing that had sat on my shelf for ages finally got opened—and read! As I devoured their pages, I learned that many of them spoke *directly* to the ailments I was facing with totally organic solutions. I was floored and earnestly began to try these natural alternatives to much success.

Fentanyl, a Schedule II narcotic more powerful than morphine, hadn't worked at all on my pain for years, but miraculously I learned that taking skullcap tincture in my tea *did work*—powerfully with real and positive effects.

I had taken Lamictal for a labeled "mood disorder" for eight years. It turns out Lamictal was actually suppressing my GABA, an amino acid that acts as a neurotransmitter in the nervous system and is an essential chemical for optimum brain and mood balance (we'll touch on this later). With a daily intake of GABA supplement, I found foul moods much easier to control and overcome.

Within a few weeks of coming off these potentially deadly drugs and opening myself up to alternative ways of healing, opportunities for cool jobs, perfect partners, inspiring friendships, and creative work flooded into my life. I quit my nine-to-five job unaffected: Less stressful work came to me before I even collected my last paycheck. I made friends who understood what I was going through. I took chances even though I wasn't sure if they'd work out. People I'd always admired became my friends. I was honest and up front with everyone, and I no longer felt upset if people didn't agree with me. I found natural solutions to not just some but *every* ailment I had ever taken pills for. These remedies, mind-strengthening techniques, and methods worked not just to ease my pain, balance my moods, and cure my anxieties, they seriously saved my life. They saved me from the only life I had known for eleven years: Days upon days spent in doctor's offices and desperately popping pills. With this new method, dozens of health problems were solved for me, sometimes overnight. I took my health and my life back one powerful, positive, proactive step at a time.

I can (humbly) say I have now inspired and coached countless others to do the same. I carry the tools that have allowed me to change my life, and so do you. I didn't grow up drinking green juice or traveling the world in search of God. It's possible, no matter your background, to live a healthy, vibrant, grounded life. Your past is not your destiny. These universal tools apply to all of us, and I'm so excited to share them with you in the pages of this book. Once you know how to use these tools, you can apply them to any situation and easily conquer each one of the areas in your life where you struggle.

These incredible tools have given me the opportunity to answer for myself one of the most important questions of all: "How do we create growth, purpose, and happiness in our lives and make them last in the long term?"

The Power of Your Mind and Beliefs

When we are kids we learn that if we spin around with our eyes closed or hold our breath, what we do with our body can instantly alter our mental state. These actions can even induce sickness. At an early age it's clear to most that the mind and body interact with each other. We observe the effects of alcohol on people's behavior. We can see the ramifications of hurtful words on someone's body posture and mood. We notice how we feel better when we eat certain foods rather than others. It's easy to recognize how we can inspire others with our behavior or our laughter. Although even as children we understand that the mind and body are connected, somewhere along the way we forget to harness this to reach our full potential.

Beliefs are the basis of what shapes your mindset. Beliefs can alter your state—they can empower you or depress you. Your beliefs are the difference between a mediocre life and an amazing one, and you're going to learn how to harness your beliefs in this book. You're going to learn how to stop allowing others to dictate how you feel and what you do, and to remember who you are at your core. Then you'll be able to reclaim your life and awaken your true self.

Your mind is the most powerful broadcasting machine in existence. It is more powerful than any spoken or written word, piece of art, or technological device. When used correctly, it can save your life. When used in the wrong way, your mind can hurt you more than anything or anyone else has the capability of doing. Our biology is no mistake. We're hardwired to be happy when something wonderful happens. We're predisposed to feeling dejected when life flows in a slightly different direction.

It's so effortless to be inspired for a little while and then lose our drive because we get caught up in a less enthusiastic moment. It seems easy to think that our answers lie in someone or something else—a person, a drug, a drink, or a certain experience, such as achieving a specific sum of money or number on a scale—and if we only had these things, we would have happiness. We make these assumptions without a second thought. These feelings are hardwired into us, but our personal patterns are ultimately what winds up triggering them.

Your biography is not your destiny. Your past does not dictate who you are now or who you can become.

Understanding Your Conditioning Factors

Our desires are conditioned by our needs. How we perceive the present moment has been conditioned by what we've experienced in our past. You can choose at any time to make a different choice than the one you made the last time. Making a different choice ultimately helps us to build a better future.

Your past is your conditioning factor—that is, every event in your life that has brought you to this present moment. Each one of these events has influenced how you process the here and now. They are the only reason you are reading these words in this exact moment in time. These are the choices that brought you here instead of to different pages in a different book.

You're here making the choice to better your life because of your conditioning factor. What that means in this case is that because of your past, you've chosen a direction in the present that will set you up to become a better version of yourself in the future. A wise choice, if I do say so myself.

Your past has conditioned you to react the way you do to your environment. You've learned to honk your horn in traffic. You've adapted to rewarding yourself with an extra hour of TV or drinking a glass of wine at night before bed. You've indulged in procrastination and called it entertainment. You've responded to stimuli the same way every day, day in and day out, perhaps for many years. You just may not have realized it.

Every day, every little thing that's happened in our lives becomes more important than it used to be. Although you may not realize it at the time, even our little inconsequential moments and the biggest, most epic defeats become so integral and important in shaping who we are and who we become. Our successes and our failures are equally valuable.

Often if you look back on difficult times, you'll find that your life was being orchestrated for you in the grandest way. What seems like the biggest, most devastating things that can happen to us at the time are often revealed to be some of our greatest blessings. Even when it feels like you've hit your limit, even when it feels like there's no point to struggling on, and even when life is cruelly unfair to you, events that seem like a major setback can really just be your conditioning factor. For example, a layoff at a toxic company may have led you to a much more rewarding job. Or a medical struggle might have opened the door to a meaningful new friendship and inspired lifelong, healthier habits.

When you learn how to grow from your setbacks and your conditions, you start to rapidly change your life.

Tame the Habit

Almost unbelievably, I now execute essentially the same routines every single morning that I did when I was on over a dozen different pharmaceutical drugs. However, exactly what I'm doing in my performance of these routines—and how and why I am doing them—has changed completely.

I call this *taming the habit*. Instead of bombarding my body with drugs and greasy foods first thing in the morning, I give my body something else. Now every day I take my first set of nutritional, body-boosting supplements with an organic fruit or vegetable smoothie. Often I take two or three supplements in tablet form.

The action of taking pills is identical. If you saw me perform my previous action and my current action behind an X-Ray machine, they would look not just similar but exactly the same. However, instead of swallowing something that could potentially harm my body, I now take pills full of natural minerals, herbs, and powders that truly support and heal my body. We are creatures of habit and we love our daily routines. Replacing our harmful habits with healthier habits enables us to continue the rituals we find rewarding or satisfying to give us a better chance of sticking with this new healthy lifestyle.

For example, if every evening you unwind with a glass of wine, but you know deep down that you should cut back on your alcohol consumption for your health, consider replacing that glass with a cup of your favorite herbal tea. You'll find many herbal teas that address our most common problems, like insomnia, depression, and anxiety, in the coming chapters. You will still feel that same sense of relaxation and moment to yourself that you are craving, but without the morning hangover or any harm done to your liver.

Seemingly small shifts in my daily habits have changed my life forever. Recognizing and then changing the parts of your behavior that are harming you is a fine-tuned skill, and you'll learn how to hone it with every page of this book.

Today, the pills I incorporate into my life are powerful vitamins, herbal tonics, and organic supplements, and they have cured me of everything from cystic acne to bad moods. They are the answer I was always looking for. I am so happy to be able to share the specific methods, techniques, and mind-strengthening tools with you throughout this book that you can use to transform your life.

You too will learn how to recognize, name, and tame your harmful habits. You can unlock the real miracles hiding in your mind, unleash your true power, and change your life for the better by implementing the WILD habits tools and techniques.

Become Your Best Self

Most people want happiness, but it's only those who remain committed to improvement that ever actually find it. You can harness your habits into a successful career, a beautiful family, or a platform to teach, inspire, and lead your community. You can turn your habits into the reason for your happiness.

If we let them, our habits can and *will* change us. If we're open, ready, and willing, we don't have to change everything. It's easy. Only a few small tweaks in our day could improve our life experience. When we harness our choices, we begin to take control of our lives.

I wasn't born depressed—I *learned* how to be depressed. Then I meticulously incorporated depression into every area of my identity. I believed the labels others had given me, and the more I focused on them, the more depressed I felt. I attracted depressed people. I listened to depressing songs. I surrounded myself with depressing objects. I gave these negative feelings my full attention and power over me, and so they grew. I wasn't born anxious. I was born on stimulants. Then I developed very few coping mechanisms along the way to handle trauma, stress, and anxiety.

My habits used to get me in trouble. I focused on the negative parts of my day, I indulged in self-destructive tendencies, and I surrounded myself with the wrong people. I exhibited one bad tendency after another until finally I had formed a bad pattern of behavior, an unsavory and depressive personality, and a poorly guided and mismanaged life.

Now my habits are the building blocks that have shaped my life and helped me grow. They're responsible for every business achievement, good word, kind person, amazing interaction, and my personal health and mental well-being. I learned how to replace my harmful habits with WILD habits. WILD habits support our positive growth and commitment to change for the better, and I will introduce them to you in this book. My WILD habits are the reason that day in and day out, I can feel secure, successful, nurtured, grateful, and content. They are the reason I have remained free of pharmaceutical drugs for seven years without ever turning back. They're the reason that I can face any problem that comes my way head on, usually with a creative, easy solution. They include mindfulness, utilizing positive energy, meditating, incorporating healing foods into my diet, fitness, natural remedies, vitamins and supplements, finding my inner purpose, and so much more. They're why my internal vision of myself matches my external body. My habits are the reason that every time I wake up, I start the day with that elusive feeling I always used to strive for: happiness.

I want that for you—every single day. I don't want you to question the best version of yourself, *I want you to be that person.* Ultimately this book will challenge you to explore your personal tendencies and to identify how they might be affecting your life. This is not about getting rid of your habits; it's about turning them into WILD habits. This book is about learning what your patterns are, and then discovering how to harness them and use them to your advantage in your life, your career, and your relationships.

You can begin to form your habits consciously instead of unconsciously. Rather than feeling like you are powerless to events or circumstances outside of yourself, you can begin to feel calm, centered, and in total control of how things play out for you. I believe you will finish this book as a better version of yourself, and I am so excited for you! This is when the real fun begins.

Real effects include having an awesome day, taking more walks, checking yourself out in the mirror, making self-loving decisions, becoming inspired, and getting your life back.

What are you waiting for? Let's get started!

PART 1

WILD SPIRIT

CHAPTER 1

My WILD Story

I watched my mother battle with an unforgiving drug and alcohol addiction, up close and personal, for the first formative years of my life. Some days she'd load me in the car and drive drunk and high to her ex-boyfriend's house. There, we'd wait all day for him to come home from work, just so that she could see the look on his face when he realized that his tires were slashed. Other days she'd take me to Taco Bell and start screaming at the staff because she was not handed a burger from Burger King. It was embarrassing at best and frightening at worst.

By the time that I was in the first grade, I had seen my mother black out on vodka and overdose on heroin countless times. The normalcy most children expect was overshadowed by the crippling effects of drugs and alcohol. I was overcome by the fear that one day—probably one day very soon—my mom wouldn't wake up anymore.

It was clear to me that my mom didn't seem to *want* to wake up anymore. She rarely woke up before 11:00 a.m.—and that was on a good day. She started forgetting to drop me off at school in the morning, and she never remembered to pick me up from after-school. I missed more than twenty days of first grade simply because Momma was hungover.

The first time I remember my mom shooting heroin was at my great aunt's funeral when I was four years old. She sequestered me in the bathroom with her and laid down in the handicapped stall.

I watched her little ritual: the powder, the lighter, the spoon, the needle, and the Big Nod, where her eyes would glaze over and I'd lose her. As a child, it seemed like she was lost for eternity.

The last time I saw my mom shooting heroin was at six years old. I climbed on top of the bed we shared. The mattress was filled with rough cigarette burns and I was wary about waking her, but it had been too long and I was hungry.

A dark chill washed over me when I couldn't rouse her at all. Her eyes were rolled in the back of her head. I didn't know the word "overdose," but I knew that she was not waking up. I tried shaking her, calling to her, and finally ran to the kitchen, pulled out a kitchen stool, and climbed on it to reach the phone.

Without the call I made to my grandparents that night, my mom would surely not be here today.

My only set of grandparents, my mom's parents, applied for custody of me after this incident. It's difficult to get custody of a child when she still has one parent left in the picture, and my bond with my mother was strong. I would have done anything for her—and often did. However, the judge granted custody of me to my grandparents at the age of seven. Maybe it was because of my honesty when I told the judge that, yes, I often walked to get my mother cigarettes alone. No, I didn't mind. It was only a mile away. The gas station guy always gave me a lollipop, too, on my way out. Or maybe it was the fact that Mom came to court wasted.

Finally, I was officially theirs. Grandma and Grandpa brought me up with the unwavering hope that my mother would eventually get sober and be able to raise me herself one day. They sent me to talk therapy immediately and were loving, guiding, and supportive.

They told me every single day, "You're somebody. You're smart; you're going to go to college and make something of your life. You will never do drugs. You will not become your mother."

While I never did do the drugs my grandparents were so worried about, by the time I was twenty-four, I was on fourteen different legal prescription drugs. And they nearly killed me.

A Chaotic Childhood

Though I thrived with my sweet grandma and grandpa, my childhood had a melancholy, chaotic, and dramatic undertone. It seemed that I could not go a single day without being confronted by daunting situations that were completely out of my control. My mother was in and out of rehab and jail. Every week I had to decide whether to read her inpatient, 12-step letters or take the phone calls that started with an automated message stating which prison was calling.

Mom was never stable. While she had been on and off cocaine and shooting heroin for years, alcohol and cigarettes were her worst addictions. She always had a Newport 100 between her fingers and a gallon of vodka hidden somewhere in the apartment. She never made it easy. Mom constantly pulled intoxicated stunts that left me heartbroken and bewildered.

I had a hard time adjusting to my new living situation in the second grade, and my grandparents had a challenging time acclimating to the realities of raising a brand-new child much later on in their lives. With two generations and a whole ocean between how and where they'd grown up, and how and where I did, this wasn't necessarily surprising. But it was lonely and alienating. It made me deeply unhappy that no one seemed to pick up on or understand the things that I understood. My grandma, for instance, used to ask me as a little kid if I thought my mother was drunk during the times we communicated when she was not in jail. I could always (and often) pick up on whether Mom was intoxicated within a few, short, desperately-trying-not-to-sound-slurred words. I could tell by her deep breaths. I could tell by how long she took to answer a question. Although my mom was awful at hiding it, my grandma always said she couldn't tell at all. There were things that I could see with ease that both my grandma and grandpa seemed oblivious to.

Most of my solace came in the form of books, music, and school, which I loved. Friends, teachers, family, counselors, strangers, and my therapist, who I started seeing at the age of seven, made daily assumptions about my capabilities based on my family history and my past. For the most part, I internalized their assumptions without much thought or review. You don't question whether your caretakers have your best interests at heart. You just assume they do.

My grandfather, who I call Dad, was loving. Though he worked full-time, Dad instantly became heavily involved in my life, driving me to rehearsals, soccer practice, dance lessons, voice lessons, and piano. Grandma was sweet and caring. A stay-at-home mom by nature, Grandma was most comfortable behind a story book and the stove. As Irish Catholic immigrants, it was not a question to my grandparents whether I would go to Catholic school, attend college, and graduate. Those were givens, as long as they kept me off drugs. Because of my past and their tough-love culture, they had higher standards for me than they'd had for their own children or even themselves. I was told every single day that I could never touch alcohol or drugs or my life would be over forever. I believed it. No one had to tell me this even twice: I had already seen firsthand how alcohol and hard drugs ruin someone's life.

Their determination was instilled in me. I was so desperate to prove to everyone that I was NOT my mother. I never missed a day of school, never skipped, and never drifted in class. I received straight A's, attended weekly therapy and Alateen meetings (hour-long meetings for the children of alcoholics), and sang at multiple church masses every weekend. I had no intention of ever touching alcohol or drugs.

I longed for my own happy ending, but as time went on, I could never seem to see it. Instead of normal childhood dreams, I suffered from severe insomnia, nightmares, and frequent panic attacks. I was haunted by the very real thought of burying my mother. My happy ending felt like it belonged to someone else, as if I were doomed to a life that was a knockoff of a Shakespearean tragedy.

The stigma of a broken and unusual family situation became more real as time passed and the gravity of my situation sunk in. My hope shrank each day. It seemed impossible that my mother would ever get well and be able to raise me. It seemed like a far-off dream that she never realized would require her to actually *do* something to achieve. If she couldn't get her act together for her one and only kid, who could she do it for? I thought to myself, *I'm clearly not enough to inspire anyone to change their life.*

Man, was I wrong.

My First "Diagnosis"

Alcoholism is often referred to as a family disease, as it affects not only the alcoholic but also has a dramatic impact on the lives of everyone who's close to them. The home life of an alcoholic family ranges from dysfunctional and erratic to severely abusive, and children within these homes develop personality traits and behaviors that are often based on their traumatic experiences in this environment.

My mother went away and got sober at an inpatient facility for a year, the longest she had been able to keep it together during my life. When she left the facility, my grandparents let my mother move in with us for a "short period of time," which turned into almost two years.

After less than twenty-four months of living with us, and only weeks away from earning my grandparents' trust forever, my mother relapsed in front of me once again—the summer right before I was to start high school. The details of my mother's relapse can be found in detail in my first book, *Cured by Nature*. Needless to say, it was traumatizing for me to experience this kind of behavior from her all over again, and I expressed that vehemently to anyone who would listen. I was so angry and heartbroken. Two years of hard work, of opening up, of letting her in . . . and I felt we were all back at square one. If I couldn't trust my own mother, how could I ever trust anyone again? *It's not fair, it's not fair, it's not fair* was my daily mantra.

This incident prompted my grandparents to send me to a child psychiatrist for the first time at the age of thirteen. After years of talk therapy, someone had suggested to them that maybe—just maybe—putting me on medication might help me "deal with" all the messed up, disorderly scenes and circumstances that had dominated my entire life so far.

A few questions, a short family history questionnaire, and mere minutes later, I had my first diagnosis: manic depression, commonly known today as bipolar disorder. This is characterized by manic highs and deep, depressive lows. I didn't feel that I had either of those things, just a gnarly case of Shitty Life Disorder. In fact, I exhibited almost no symptoms of my diagnosis. I had never been on a "manic high," there was no money for me to recklessly spend, my mood was relatively predictable, I had never been paranoid, I had no issues at school— behavioral or otherwise—I suffered from no delusions, and I only felt depressed when something out of my control happened. Who, put in my situation, wouldn't be at least a little bit depressed?

My first heavy-duty pharmaceutical medication was prescribed to me that very day, at the age of thirteen. It was a mood stabilizer called lithium. At the time, it was a Band-Aid meant to mask the trauma of watching my mother relapse in front of me, time and time again.

Antipsychotic drugs like lithium are meant to be taken for life. If you protest, doctors call that a "symptom of your illness" and will often prescribe you more or alternative medication. They might even threaten to commit you to a mental hospital. They tried all of these things with me any time I questioned what I was taking or why.

I took lithium exactly as it was prescribed to me. Every morning, 1,500 milligrams (three 500 milligram pills). I didn't have a choice. On day one my grandma told me, "If you don't take this, you can't go to school." That was the ultimate threat for me. I absolutely loved school.

After a few weeks, I could see that it was working. I felt like a complete zombie. My brain slowed down—it took me longer to read a page or finish a book. It also took me longer to grasp a concept in class or to understand the point a friend was making to me in a personal story. But strangely, it did not make what I had witnessed in my life any better or easier to digest. These memories still haunted me, and perhaps even more so, as I did not have the mental clarity anymore to deal with them. I was angry underneath the surface, but all I could express was complete ennui. I went from feeling angry and sad to feeling literally nothing.

Not only did lithium not make my trauma any better, it also changed me almost entirely. My brain came to a complete halt, and unexpectedly my whole body slowed down, too. I got incredibly weak, a side effect of lithium now called asthenia. I could barely lift a jar off the table. I had a hard time with sports like soccer, which I had loved before. After every game, I was completely breathless. More than that, I had a hard time concentrating. For the first time ever, I had to read one page in a book two or three times to understand it.

Even when I tried to deal with my feelings, conjuring up any inspiration to face them felt like too large a task. A new feeling dominated them all. I called this the Empty Feeling, which haunted me for over a decade. This feeling started only *after* I began taking lithium, a drug meant to address feelings of sadness, emptiness, and despair.

This was my first drug, my first label, and the first time I started to feel powerless. Now, no matter how much I protested, I was always met with the largest wall of all: mental illness. "Now Tara, you know what the doctor says," was the familiar comeback, no matter what the issue. It was constantly held over my head. After my diagnosis, any of my future suggestions for my own mental or physical wellbeing were totally dismissed.

The true reach of a mental illness label's stigma, and the subsequent effect that one diagnosis could have on a life, were completely unimaginable to me at the time.

More Diagnoses—and More Prescriptions

I loved school because I was good at it. Grade school into high school, I was a straight-A student and had (somehow, miraculously) never drifted mentally in class—not even for a few moments. Distraction was not a word I was familiar with. When I put my mind to something, it always got done. I loved learning to a dorky degree. I did my homework early; I read the entire textbook before we officially started the school year, and I spent all my free time at the library.

After about twenty months on lithium, school became more difficult. My grades in math, foreign language, and science began to slip, and I had trouble concentrating. I experienced brain fog for the first time ever. It felt like I was swimming in murky thoughts. Twice, I brought home a C+ on a test, which was incredibly out of character for me. Worse, it spelled trouble for First Honors, a list on which my name was proudly printed every semester since sixth grade.

Immediately, my grandparents called the doctor. Something was wrong with me, they insisted. They were taking me in!

My psychiatrist looked disappointed. It didn't take long for him to identify this grave disorder that had brought two C+'s into my life: Attention Deficit Hyperactivity Disorder. I'd never heard of it before.

My diagnosis was in 2003. Today, ADHD is one of the most common diagnoses in the United States for kids. The CDC has claimed that it affects roughly 11 percent of all American children ages four to seventeen.

Immediately, I was placed on a medication called Metadate CD, which is now commonly prescribed for children as young as five. The more I thought about it, the more I didn't quite understand this diagnosis. Even the name, Attention Deficit. Hyperactivity. Disorder. It didn't have a single word in it that resonated with me. I definitely wasn't attention deficit or hyperactive. But once again, I didn't have a choice. I had to take this medication every day before school—and I never refused. Metadate's side effects include: vision problems; dizziness; mild headache; stomach pain, nausea, and vomiting; loss of appetite; numbness, tingling, and cold feelings in your hands or feet; nervous feelings; and sleep problems. I had them all.

A few weeks after starting Metadate was, ironically, the first time in my life that my entire GPA had ever begun to decline. I went from straight A's to C's and sometimes even D's in math, foreign language, and science. I was baffled. Wasn't this medication supposed to help me do better?

I was wired. I bombed at singing auditions, nearly my sole comfort and source of self-esteem. I shook constantly, I developed a small twitch, and my appetite disappeared. My tiny frame lost one too many pounds, and my grandparents noticed. I'd bless people in the name of Jesus Christ, their cat from Venus that they had three lives ago, and walk away.

After a few weeks and a little defiance, I was taken off Metadate. At this time, my psychiatrist also informed me that lithium might just be inhibiting my learning abilities. I asked him what he meant by that.

"It can," he explained, "make it hard for some kids to do math, learn other languages, and grasp science. It's okay, it's okay. We'll switch it."

I was livid, and it must have showed. First of all, why wasn't I told this before I was put on another drug to address the poor grades? Second, *why wasn't I told this in the first place?!*

I was switched from lithium to a drug called Lamictal, which is used for seizures, clinical depression, mania, and mood disorders. It made me feel a little less zombie-like than lithium, but it had strange side effects. My doctor said that if I ever developed a rash to call him immediately. A Lamictal rash can lead to a skin condition that will kill you.

Despite this concern, my dosage was constantly increased and tweaked. I didn't want to try a different drug, so I just stopped complaining. When my doctor asked, I said I was fine. Feeling better. Doing better.

I wasn't.

But I stayed on Lamictal for the next eight and a half years of my life.

Physical Pain—and More Pills!

At age eleven I was diagnosed with a severe case of scoliosis, which is a painful curvature of the spine. I wore a back brace for three years (clearly I was super popular during this time!) and attended physical therapy weekly. Unfortunately, my therapist was doing my exercises backwards and had actually been making my spine much worse in the process!

I was in pain. Every. Single. Day. My back was constantly inflamed and worse, every time I saw a doctor about it, I left with a prescription for high-dose Tylenol and had wasted three hours of my life I'd never get back.

At sixteen years old, a diagnosis of juvenile rheumatoid arthritis was added to my growing list of labels. I was prescribed yet another pill each day, a muscle relaxer called Vioxx, at the age of seventeen. Vioxx was later taken off the market (for reasons we'll touch on in chapter nine). I was still in high school and kept my bottle of Vioxx in my backpack. It rattled loudly and ominously as I walked from class to class. Although I took the pills diligently, I was still in pain every single day. I finally, truly, and concretely believed I was sick. As my teens turned into my twenties, I continued to take more and more pills, which only made me feel worse and worse.

I had managed to abandon all of the coping mechanisms that therapy, family, teachers, mentors, and books had tried to impart on me in my youth. I was truly a mess—mentally, physically, emotionally, and psychologically—and I didn't know that there was another way out.

There is. But when a prescription pill doesn't help you, it often feels like there may be no other way out. Rx drugs are the first line of defense for any and all of these kinds of problems. When they don't work, it can seem like there is no other solution. This is one of the most helpless places we find ourselves, especially in this culture, where we have been so thoroughly convinced that pharmaceutical medication alone is the number one solution to our health problems.

The (Not So) Prime of My Life

I felt completely helpless in my body and mind. I had lost more than a handful of friends at an early age to various tragedies, including drug overdoses and suicide. In my first year at college, five classmates passed away. It felt like death was following me.

I had been in nothing but toxic relationships, including a physically and emotionally abusive relationship (for three miserable years) with someone who tried to kill me. I had been to more funerals for friends and loved ones than I cared to count. With an alcoholic and opiate-addicted parent in and out of the picture, and the other biological parent out of the picture entirely, I had seen more messed up things than I ever wanted to sit down and tell a therapist—or even a friend—about.

Although I had a good, stable job working in a laboratory at Cornell, it involved long hours indoors, and I was deeply unhappy. I longed for real happiness. I wanted to feel excited to wake up in the morning. I wanted to have to tone down my thrill for life. I could feel strings in the cosmos tugging at me, reminding me, "Be here now." I wanted to be floored by my own existence and share the knowledge of life's intricacies with the people I knew most needed to hear it. I wrote long poems, free-form thought pieces, and diary entries at night about my connection to the patchwork of humanity. I felt what others felt, and I wanted a way to make it better for everyone.

Most people see a doctor when they get sick, not when they get well. We are encouraged to consult a doctor when something is wrong, but we're not encouraged in the same way to explain to a doctor when, if, or how we've recovered on our own. I watched throngs of people come through the doors of Cornell because they were sick; I saw almost no one come in because they felt better. I noticed that most people, if they've made it to a doctor's appointment at all, are completely at their wit's end.

I noticed distinct patterns in patient's self-care and harmful habits (many of which I'll be touching on in this book), which had led them down different but equally troubling paths of body-mind destruction. They were disconnected from themselves, from nature, and from their bond with others. They were plugged in and tuned out. They were often so caught up in their tasks that they had forgotten the true point of what they were doing. I would watch patients, doctors, surgeons, nurses, business meetings and interpersonal work relationships begin with one point and end on another, never solving the core root of the problem. I saw the sunken faces of people who were dissatisfied patrons of their own lives. I saw clearly the unhealthy habits that had led to unhealthy people. Each day, I noticed the same patterns in myself, too. But like many of the desperate folks I watched walk through our doors, I felt helpless to stop these patterns in myself. They seemed much easier to recognize in other people.

I watched two summers go by from the twenty-seventh floor window of the lab. I felt like a part of me was fading away every day as I missed the opportunity to let any of those sunrays hit my face. Was there any way out of this mess? There was. Many of my answers were right in front of me. But I was too busy coasting on other people's ideas of what my life should be. I was striving for someone else's version of success—a job (with benefits, of course!), a relationship, and a family. I was deeply in the fog of over a dozen pills, which had been swimming throughout my body for as long as I could remember. With empty, unfulfilled promises attached to swallowing every single one of them, thousands of times over, it was getting hard to see what "help" truly looked like. I was becoming not just sick and tired, but a dangerous counterpart—I was becoming hopeless and helpless.

At the break of day my eyes opened, and I was hit with the Empty Feeling in the pit of my stomach. Every single morning the very first thing I did was take a pill (or five) that promised to make it go away. The pills sometimes numbed me out, put me to sleep, or painted over my reality with a milky brush, but they never delivered the help I was searching for. They never made things better. They never brought me a feeling of happiness or euphoria. They never handed over the manageable, pain-free life that they had pinky promised. Additionally, after many years of this daily drug use, I needed more of the same drug to experience similar effects.

Often I was too ashamed to admit that many of these pharmaceuticals didn't seem to be working at all. As in, not even a little bit. *Horrifying*, I thought. *What's wrong with me that even fentanyl, a narcotic fifty to a hundred times more powerful than morphine, doesn't take my pain away?*

In fact, many of the drugs I took even had adverse or augmented effects, such as increased pain, muscle spasms, extreme weight loss, and mood swings. Be that as it may, a doctor had told me that this was my answer, so for more than a decade, every single time I felt an emotion, sensation, or pain that I was uncomfortable with, I took the pill that they had told me to take.

Hitting Rock Bottom

To others, I was a bright, well-employed, glowing, young woman with a wicked sense of humor and an unshakable spirit. No matter what kind of day I was having, no matter how shitty I felt, no matter what medication I was taking, I still managed to make everyone around me smile. I had a mess of raven curls down my back, a splatter of freckles across my nose, and a desire to change the world for the better. But behind it all I was hiding a miserable interior that was begging for understanding and release. I desperately wanted the feeling of comfort—the kind of comfort that comes with waking up healthy and happy.

I was twenty-four, and a few weeks earlier I had gone to the funeral of one of my best friends, Grey, who had been my age. Life felt strange, foreign, and empty without her. Her suicide had torn apart my entire group of friends. With my support system gone and an abusive relationship with a boyfriend at its peak, I was lost. This was definitely rock bottom for me.

I grieved in selfish ways: I pushed people away, I drank, I took more pills than I was supposed to, and, ultimately, I got put on the regimen of drugs that truly put me over the edge. Valium and Xanax had been added to my daily dosages of painkillers, mood stabilizers, antidepressants, birth control, muscle relaxers, nerve blockers, and . . . I truly lost it. My thoughts were murky, selfish, and terribly dark. I might have looked happy some of the time, but I secretly hated myself almost all of the time.

On top of this, I believed that bad luck followed me, that I was a mistake and therefore doomed to be unlucky and to always be alone and unloved. I was convinced that life had dealt me a bad hand and that being lonely was the worst thing in the whole world. I felt that I was broken, unstable, and inherently emotionally sensitive. I felt called to do something radical.

This helpless, powerless feeling is what culminated in my own suicide attempt in March 2011. I opened up my entire left arm with a razor blade I had stolen from work. My memories are hazy and underwater. My eyes welled up with tears, but I could barely cry.

My boyfriend at the time—the abusive control freak who was completely toxic for me—showed up at my apartment just in time. He was shocked at the sight of my arm and appalled at the reality of my choice. We were mid-fight, and he was the last person I expected to swoop in and decide to become my guardian angel for the night. He started crying, quietly asking me over and over again, "Tara, what did you do? *What did you do?*"

I watched him begin to apply gauze and wrap my wounds to stop the bleeding. I watched the blood pool and soak through the gauze, and I was so, so disappointed. I had expected a release. A euphoria. A rush. I realized that instead I felt nothing. Numb. Shit. Zero. Zilch. Nothing. Absolutely nothing had changed.

I realized then that I didn't really want to die. I just wanted the feeling of emptiness to disappear.

Fortunately, my suicide attempt failed, and when I couldn't feel any pain I recognized that something radical needed to happen—and it wasn't taking my own life. I saw, finally, that nearly everything in my life needed to change. I didn't want to simply be alive; I wanted to be living my wildest dreams. I suddenly realized what I'd lose if I went down that route. I looked down at my arm and truly saw myself for the first time ever. In the messiest, lowest time in my life, I finally saw that there was *nothing wrong with me*. I was perfect, divine, and most of all: human. Being human meant I was smart enough, capable enough, and intelligent enough to know that I had a choice. Awful things had happened to me, but only *I* chose how to handle them. And I didn't need to handle them by doing more fucked up things to myself. That had never solved anything, and it never would.

My beliefs were the sole reason I had done this to myself. Powerless beliefs had led to powerless convictions. Powerless convictions had led to what humans inevitably do next when they're desperate: drastic, dramatic, powerless actions. The only way to prevent these actions from happening in the future was to make sure that my beliefs were different.

The only way I could handle the future was to be better next time. If I could be better every day, if I could make a different choice, if I could see a perfect person behind all my scars and all my trauma, then maybe I could get better. And if I knew how to get better, then

I could truly *be* better—permanently and in the long run. That's why I had taken pills for so long: I wanted to *be* better. If I wanted to be better, I had to act better. If I wanted to act better, I had to think better. If I wanted to think better, I probably shouldn't be on fourteen different drugs.

This is what ultimately solidified my decision to come off my Rx meds—cold turkey. I just woke up and decided I was done. I broke up with my boyfriend, cut out all my toxic relationships, told a few people to get lost, and started over. Clean slate, I told myself. This is *it*.

The first few days, it wasn't hard at all. Other than having to stop my automatic reactions or habits (filling up a glass of water, reaching into my bag, opening a medicine cabinet), it was unbelievably easy. I thought, *I got this*. Then, I noticed it creep in.

Stopping my meds affected my vision and colors would change like I was on acid, a drug I had never even taken. I'd have to remind myself that the sky wasn't purple. That trees weren't blue. That objects were probably a little farther away than they appeared to be. After week one, the withdrawal became aggressive. It started with dizziness. The room would begin spinning, and I felt like someone was standing on me after spinning me around. I could hardly stand up for more than a few minutes and was always breathless. Every single shower was spent sitting down with my head tucked in between my knees. Then came the shakes and tremors, where I could not hold a glass of water and often stuck my head under the shower to drink from there. I could no longer eat, but I had an uncontrollable hunger in my belly. I experienced brain zaps, missed periods, and two-month-long periods.

After a few weeks, I realized that this decision could kill me. I do not recommend coming off prescription medications cold turkey. This is my honest experience, but **don't do it**. If I could go back and change it, I would. I was desperately in need of an IV and several doctors. Taking out your own vomit baskets curbside is not as glamorous as they make it look in movies or reality television. There is no makeup girl to come and powder your face. No one tells you you'll wake up in wet sheets from your own sweat. No one warns you what bile smells like coming out of your mouth. I carried tissues with me because my nose was always clogged after throwing up. I inhaled the stale taste of vomit every time I took a breath. I didn't sleep a single night straight for many months. I used a bedpan because I was bedridden.

Brain fog became my new normal. I would look down at a table and say *fork, fork, fork* to myself over and over, but I couldn't, for the life of me, actually pick out which item was the fork. My work suffered. My relationships changed rapidly. It was finally time. I was purging everything.

Living My Best Life

When I thought about meeting my needs, I was reminded of my suicide attempt every day for many months. My wounds stung and needed to be properly cleaned and dressed every day.

I still remember the epiphany I had one night in the tiny bathroom of my New York apartment. I was changing my dressing and nursing my fresh wounds. Staring at one of the larger wounds, I suddenly realized how selfish my actions had been. I realized how absolutely silly it was of me to think that my problems would somehow end with death. I realized that what we call problems are merely life lessons—much like my actions here had been. These wounds had become a reminder to never treat myself this way again. To be more loving. To be more caring. To treat myself like I had hoped for so long that other people would treat me: with care and respect.

I decided that I was going to conquer the hopeless feeling that had plagued me all my life. When my suicide attempt failed, I couldn't deny that my life had been spared for a reason. When all signs had pointed to NO, a force outside of myself had said YES. Did I want to continue on my current path to stay miserable, or did I want to be happy? It didn't seem like a hard choice anymore. I had been given a second chance. For once, I had the opportunity to start over. I was determined not to waste it.

What we call problems are both larger and smaller than the physical world. They're the greatest teachers we have, and they teach the most inspiring lessons. Negative experiences may happen to you or around you, but you're the one who has to choose how to respond to them. Are you going to tailgate the person who cut you off or send him or her a loving prayer? Are you going to run away from your problems or face them? Are you going to turn your hardest challenges into your greatest lessons?

A lot of negative things had happened to me, but only *I* had chosen to hurt myself this time. And only I could choose to be better, stronger, and more fearless next time. This was my first major lesson in abandoning judgment and finding gratitude. Instead of hating or resenting these deep wounds, I accepted—without judgment—that I would very likely live with these scars for life. I was finding a way, each and every day, to feel grateful for them. As I dressed and cleaned my wounds every morning and evening, I began to see each long mark over my veins as a warrior tattoo: a sign of inner strength. I had gone into battle completely fearless and had come out the other side bruised, battered, and scarred but enlightened. I had fought the greatest battle in the world—the war with myself. And I had won.

Through that experience and realization, I finally got the very thing I had always wanted. I received the one radical shift that I had always sought the most: I got rid of the Empty Feeling for good. It was in that moment when I sat in gratitude that I really got inspired and excited for the first time since I was a child. I realized that nothing and no one was going to change for me. If I wanted to see change in my life, I was the one who had to change my life. And having that power was incredible. I didn't have to rely on anyone else to solve my problems for me—I was going to do that now, and I was motivated to start. I had to face my toxic choices, my unhealthy relationships, and my thoughtless dependencies. My brain lit up with ideas and creative solutions almost immediately. I had the power to choose how deep my next breath was, what direction my next step would be, and, ultimately, what path my life would take, if only I was open to making a more conscious shift. I was ready, willing, and open to making this radical change. I was ready to have a better life experience. Better than ready, I was committed to getting better and being healthy, as well as finding personal accomplishment and success. It turns out that commitment was the framework that I had been missing all along on my way to building the foundation of my life.

In these inspired, motivational moments of clarity, we are feeling pure self-acceptance and self-love. These are the "aha" moments when we can finally envision a future, and it looks a lot different from our present. I had a commitment to happiness because I finally felt like I deserved to be happy. I was done with being a victim. I didn't want to WANT a better life, I wanted to LIVE a better life.

The feeling that I had to do something radical remained, but the feeling that this radical action should be negative disappeared entirely. I knew that I had wasted too much time already doing the wrong things, trying to please the wrong people, acting out for the wrong reasons. Pain, both emotional and physical, had haunted me as a cruel memory. For as long as I could recall, I had masked it with more doctor's visits, more pills, and more prescriptions. It was legal and easy, but it hadn't worked.

I knew that I had it in me to change completely, but people had tried to change me all my life with no success. Pills hadn't worked. Therapy hadn't worked. The worst possible life circumstances had changed nothing. Based on this, I knew that change had to start with one important person.

Me.

I quit my secure job about a month after the symptoms of withdrawal began. Once the weakness, brain fog, sweating, and bone and muscle pain started, I knew it wasn't safe to continue to work. The same week that I quit, I started fighting racing thoughts, insomnia, and extreme vomiting and nausea. I lived off of my meager savings and unemployment benefits while trying to figure out what my next steps would be.

I couldn't do much. No one tells you how bad it's going to feel. Withdrawal was disgusting in ways I could never have imagined. Giving up pharmaceutical medication meant, in essence, giving up control of my whole body. I no longer chose when or if I could sit up. I had no say over the dizziness. I had no control over the brain fog, the shakes, the stomach cramps, or the extreme vomiting and dehydration. Suddenly I'd break out into a cold sweat, and I knew it was coming; I'd make a break for the nearest bathroom. Soon, I couldn't even do that. As I went through it, I found I was severely struggling to get out of bed in the morning. Every day I grew weaker and more frail. Every morning my throat was raw from throwing up the night before. I often woke up dry heaving, which made me scared to fall asleep. I didn't want to choke on my own vomit and die. This had happened to more than one of my mother's AA comrades after a blackout and had made it up there with some of my worst nightmares ever.

I had a very small support system and mostly went through withdrawal on my own. I didn't tell my family what I was doing for a myriad of reasons. First of all, I didn't want them to feel guilty about putting me on medication to begin with, because this wasn't about them. I knew they were only doing what they felt was best for me in their eyes. This was about doing what was best for me in *my* eyes. Remember, at the time my goal was to find out what medication I "needed" and what medication I did not need. The goal was not to stay off all my Rx drugs forever. That came later, when I realized that so many natural alternatives out there actually worked. I only told a handful of people that I had come off my Rx drugs, and even that ended up being mostly a mistake, because the majority of the people in my life generally had a completely negative influence on me.

My destructive ex-friends tried to discourage any and all of my healthy behaviors, which I realize now is common. I was attracted to these people when I had been sick, not when I was well. They were used to me being the one who was always at the doctor's office, purse rattling with pills they could plunder when my back was turned. And they didn't like the idea of me getting better.

I didn't even have a support system in my former colleagues. I tried to see doctors about my withdrawals a handful of times, but I was met with three distinct options:

1. Check myself into the hospital, which was most likely the safest route but did not make sense for me financially or personally at the time, since I didn't have great health insurance and lived alone with my dog, who had no alternate caretaker. (I also figured it was likely their solution at a hospital would be to administer drugs.)

2. Go back on medication and slowly wean myself off again under doctor supervision (which made the least sense to me logically since I had already come so far).

3. Go on different medication (which wasn't the point).

When I wouldn't take their drugs or check into their hospital, all my doctors just shrugged and told me to please, please be careful if I insisted on doing this at home. They each had a "you'll be back and I'll say I told you so" look on their face. I found out why. My nausea got so bad that it was constant. Sweats, chills, brain fog, dehydration, abdominal pain, migraines, inflammation, shakes, extreme vomiting, night terrors, brain zaps. It was unbearable. Like having ten flus, the worst hangover of your life, and coming off heroin—all at once. I was afraid to fall asleep at night; I prayed and pictured a day where I'd have complete control again. Where I could choose when I'd get up, if I'd leave the house, and where I would go.

My Happy Place

My happy place is a feeling: the feeling of freedom. And I will never take that for granted. Your happy place doesn't have to be a place; it can be a connection to your body, a stretch you start your morning with, a return smile from a stranger, or a light in your eyes. I prayed for the day when I'd know what it was all for, and that day came sooner than I ever could have imagined.

Books that taught me how to meditate, celebrate life, begin a gratitude practice, or find natural alternatives to the drugs I had taken for years all fell into my lap, just when I needed to read them. They had been sitting on my bookshelf for years, and then overnight I *truly saw them.* Then, I picked them up and read them. It didn't take me long to find answers and solutions to problems that had plagued me for decades.

Suddenly, people came into my life exactly when it made sense to meet them. Alternatives to my issues came to light. Circumstances aligned for me to road trip from New York to California, the perfect place for my health and the ideal way to begin my adventure and clean slate. I wrote every day. I opened my heart up wide and concentrated on people who meant the most to me: my family, my lifelong friends and my new acquaintances, who were proving to be surprisingly supportive and loyal.

Phone calls I'd been praying for came in every few days with new and exciting opportunities to live a life I had only dreamed of months before. I thought more optimistically, I trusted my gut, and I treated myself with respect. I began to feel better. I found a strength inside myself I was not previously aware that I had. And even though I still suffered from symptoms of withdrawal that were hard to get through, after a few months they subsided enough so that I could start taking actions toward making my dreams become more than dreams.

As I found solutions to some of my ailments and watched myself get a little healthier every day, I began to find myself with opportunities for projects I had prayed for my whole life. For instance, within just weeks of coming off my Rx drugs, I received a phone call from my agent, whom I hadn't heard from in about six months. I had turned her down for everything, first because of my 9-5 job, and later my reason was that I was so sick from my withdrawal symptoms.

"Betty, I'm bedridden," I had told her the last time.

"One day we'll find you a job that gets you out of bed," She told me. She thought I was exaggerating—a lazy millennial model who didn't want to work. If only she knew. I was throwing up fifteen times a day!

But this time when she called, I couldn't say no. She rang me up with the opportunity of a lifetime and an additional bonus: I had about six weeks to get healthier before we started shooting!

I signed on to act in a major motion picture. Though it was a bit part, I still spent time on set with Mark Ruffalo and chatted up

Stuart Blumberg, the Oscar-nominated director. This truly reignited my passion for a craft I had all but abandoned since college. I would often get sick on my way to set, but once there, could keep it together for the hour or so that they needed me on camera. There was something therapeutic about it, too. It energized me.

That same month, I started a band (for the first time since sixth grade!) and I took actions towards my goals every week: showing up to record, write, rehearse or brainstorm, even during some of my worst withdrawal periods. Yes, I needed to know where the nearest bathroom was at all times, but I was moving forward. I wasn't healthy by any means, but I was showing up. And I had made the most important shift of all. I was changing my habits.

Once I started acting on the inspiration that I had to get better, I *felt* better. Like flipping a switch, I went from feeling better temporarily to understanding that I was truly *getting better permanently*! It was the most uncomfortable time in my life, and I was my happiest. Truly glowing. That's when I realized that the theory I had of how to get better was no longer a theory. I had proof that it concretely and undoubtedly *worked*. I was getting better every day because I kept making different, better choices. I had seen a perfect, divine, healthy person behind all my labels and trauma, and I knew that I could become that person and reflect that image of myself out into the world. Once I knew *how* to get better, I knew that I could truly *be* better. Instead of relying on the route already laid out for me, one that had never truly worked, I now relied on constant self-improvement as my only focus. Abandoning all the noise of unnecessary medication, bad habits, and destructive relationships, and instead focusing on constant self-improvement and my core passions, had truly worked. On top of really feeling better every day, I also had hope—a key ingredient that had been missing from my life for a long, long time.

Miraculously, since making my radical shift seven years ago, I have not only successfully come off all my unnecessary meds without ever turning back, but have also been able to drop all my chronic diagnoses and labels. I still occasionally suffer from the inflammation associated with arthritis, but my depression, anxiety, mood swings, precancerous cells, hormonal issues, cystic acne, fibromyalgia, ADHD, self-harm behavior, anemia, suicidal thoughts, daily pain, chronic infections, and more have all disappeared completely and on a long-term basis. *And I haven't taken a single pharmaceutical drug for any of them.*

I cannot imagine a life filled with the sadness, disease (dis-ease), and misery I was used to for the twenty-four years before this shift, but I *can* see how easy it is to get caught up in. I watch others succumb to the same powerless feelings that I used to have every day, and I know that now I'm here as a resource to help them.

Free from that daily haunting feeling, I moved to California and took my life and my health back. Since making the commitment to my health, I've conquered my bad habits. By focusing on self-improvement, I've grown an award-winning business in a company and blog, The Organic Life, which began as a way to share my health journey with others.

At first I was so timid to share that I had taken so many new-concept, alternative routes for my health. New Yorkers are *really* not into woo-woo shit. Everyone knew I was on drugs—what would people think when they learned I'd come off of them? Would someone label this as one long "manic episode" and dismiss all the hard work I had put in? Would people discourage me on a mass scale?

The exact opposite happened. I received emails from the girls who'd teased me in high school asking how I'd come off Valium. Strangers from all over the world sent me heartfelt DMs on Twitter inquiring *exactly how much* fenugreek to take for optimum feminine health. I got emails from friends, family, and acquaintances who were reading my blogs and actually applying the articles to their lives! They wrote, "Love that organic lipstick you recommended—it performs just as well as MAC!" and "The diet and supplements you wrote about a few months back CURED my alopecia! After being bald for ten years, I have hair again! Thank you for GIVING ME MY LIFE BACK!" Some of the messages made my cry, others made me laugh out loud, but they all validated the steps I was taking to a better life. Once people saw in me—in my demeanor, my energy, my skin, my hair, my writing style, my life, my glow, my inspiration, my articles—that my route to healing was truly working, they instantly took notice.

My first book, *Cured by Nature*, hit best-seller lists right out of the gate and skyrocketed to number one in its first week. I now get to spend my days creating healthy beauty products, researching natural remedies, and connecting with folks all around the world about wellness. Through this successful platform, I have been gifted an amazing tribe of friends, readers, clients, teachers, mentors, and students. I finally understand—and very much appreciate—all of my healthy and growing relationships. I've been lucky enough to share my message globally and through some of the most respected platforms in the world.

Cured by Nature, my company, my message, and my blog have been covered by popular media outlets such as *Forbes, Teen Vogue*, Livestrong, *Glamour* magazine, *Reader's Digest, Travel + Leisure, Woman's Day*, PIX11 News, and many more. Still quite humbling to me, I was graciously honored by *San Diego Business Journal* as one of the Most Admired CEOs of 2017, as well as one of the healthiest companies of the year, and Business Woman of the Year. I also proudly display my certificate as a finalist for Woman of the Year by *San Diego Magazine* in my office—my fifth business award in less than twelve months. More than accolades to me, these awards are a reflection of hard work paying off.

However, none of these achievements are what brings me happiness. I cultivated happiness and wellness first, and then I brought happiness and wellness into everything I did. I've managed to survive, thrive, grow, teach, and learn all along the way. My businesses are now able to give back to organizations and wellness charities that mean a lot to me, a goal that has always been dear to my heart.

I now understand how temporary the pain really was. I suffered for months, but I got my *entire life* back. My temporary pain was completely worth the long-term benefits: happiness and wellness forever, and transcendence from fear. I now know why I suffered and what I was meant to learn.

It was all so that I can share this knowledge with you.

CHAPTER 2

WILD Habits

Taming my habits has made an incredible impact on the life I live today. The people who've known me the longest will be the first to tell you that I am the healthiest, happiest, and most successful I've ever been—or ever even dreamed of being—in my whole life. I have been off all pharmaceutical drugs for seven years without a single relapse. I see doctors as needed (which is once a year for a checkup, rather than every few weeks like I used to). I treat myself naturally if anything does start to pop up (which is rare) and can usually prevent an illness before it begins to manifest.

For example, I used to get the flu every year like clockwork. Each winter between January and February, I'd mentally prepare myself for the bone aches, night sweats, and solid two weeks in bed. For years, I saw this as an inevitability—a flaw in my genetics. I was, I thought, just "someone who gets the flu." When I made my natural switch, I began to use preventive medicine to battle this chronic ailment. I started by taking a calcium carbonate and probiotic shot every other morning with my breakfast. Calcium is needed by the body for healthy bones, muscles, nervous systems, and hearts, and probiotics protect the body against illness, especially those targeting your digestion and respiratory system. I also take activated charcoal internally, which absorbs and eliminates the impurities in the bloodstream that might trigger chronic illness.

I added twice daily hikes with my dogs to improve my cardiovascular system. Then I began a moderate exercise regimen at night to naturally tire me out before bed and help to regulate my circadian rhythms.

I haven't had so much as a common cold in seven years.

We choose how we rise.

Every morning for eleven years before this mental switch I woke up, turned on the sink, filled up a glass of cloudy tap water, and took a handful of pills. I was in the hospital for chronic infections almost more frequently than I was at home. The nurses at the ER knew me by name, as did my pharmacist, who had seen me weekly for over ten years. Every morning I took my pills, but I never thought about what I was doing to my body, my mind, or my spirit with this little ritual.

This same morning ritual is followed by 70 percent of Americans. That many people are on at least one pharmaceutical drug. Thirty-five percent of Americans are taking two or more Rx drugs. Antibiotics, antidepressants, and opioids are most common on the list. That's three in every five folks—all taking heavy-duty pharmaceutical drugs. And while certainly some people have mental or physical illnesses that require prescription drugs, many people self-medicate or are given medications to help with mild symptoms that could be better addressed in natural ways. If you have been diagnosed with a severe psychiatric illness, then you may indeed have a chemical imbalance that requires medication. However, if you experienced a difficult life event and were handed some Prozac or Xanax to get through it, you may want to explore new ways of managing challenging situations.

Honestly, I was never even taught that these *were* drugs. And if my grandparents ever got wind that they were powerful, addictive, adult-dosages of drugs that could have serious ramifications on my body, they NEVER would have put me on them as a young girl. They had spent countless hours and a large chunk of their savings making sure I *never* touched drugs.

Ironic? Maybe. More like bone-chillingly common. I don't blame my grandparents in the least for their decision to put me on pharmaceutical drugs as a form of therapy. After all, they had paid my psychiatrist upwards of $125 an hour to help me. What were they going to do, *not* take his advice? If my grandparents knew that there was an alternative, natural way to help me, I have no doubt they would have taken that route of treatment before ever trying antipsychotic drugs.

We are all under the delusion that we're "doing the right thing" when we fill a prescription given to us by a doctor. At no point along the way did any of the doctors who were prescribing me these pills ever ask me about my diet, my beliefs, my tendencies, my friends, or even my everyday thought patterns. They never did a blood test. They never suggested that I get a second opinion, or that I come off the drugs if they weren't working. The answer was always: more and different drugs. Granted, not every doctor so willingly prescribes drugs to treat every symptom, but we do live in a culture where medication is often the first line of defense, because it's seen as a quick fix and because most medical doctors receive very little training in nutrition or natural and alternative remedies.

Without guidance, we may never realize that our *true* quick fix lies in simple, everyday things that we're already doing: the food that we're eating, the thoughts we're thinking, the breaths that we're taking, the people that we're surrounding ourselves with. We're hardly ever taught to go within for any of our answers. In fact, we're often taught that every one of our answers lies *outside* of ourselves—in medicine, in doctors, in teachers, and in our elders. Books are written by other people. Science is discovered by someone else. We are only smart enough to blindly trust what we're told by others.

The idea that we can unlock our own health with our own minds may seem like nonsense to you. I know it used to seem that way to me, but it's true. Each one of us is capable of it. The answer to unlocking our personal power lies directly in our personal habits. A habit is defined as *a thing that you do, often and almost without thinking, especially something that is hard to stop doing.* It's repeated regularly, often subconsciously, and it's usually very difficult to quit. From the standpoint of psychology, a habit is a fixed way of thinking, willing, or feeling acquired through previous repetition of a mental experience.

Habitual behavior frequently goes unnoticed in the person exhibiting it. Since a person does not need to engage in self-analysis when undertaking routine tasks, many habits become compulsory and are repeated daily without any second thought at all. Since we do not take the time for this self-reflection, repetitive tendencies build up over many years and eventually transform into habits.

Maybe as a kid you got nervous before a test and started biting your fingernails to quell your anxiety. Today, you unconsciously gnaw at your nails when you're stressed out. You always seem to bite your nails during anxious or uncomfortable moments: in the middle of a first date or during a work presentation (the *last* times you want to be caught with this habit!). This is a small habit, but the lack of control or lack of self-esteem that it can cause may be extremely harmful to you psychologically. Nail biting may seem like an uncontrollable habit. It may feel like the only tool you have to quiet your anxiety. It may make you insecure, either consciously or subconsciously. It may instill a sense of guilt. It may seem impossible to stop. Or maybe you've even justified that it's harmless. Perhaps you've accepted this habit as a part of who you are—but it doesn't have to be!

The habits that are repeated most often, with the least benefit to us, are our harmful habits. In this chapter I will show you how to recognize your harmful habits, harness them, and transform them into WILD habits that support your best self.

Identifying Your Harmful Habits

What if you had to relearn how to drive a car every time you got in the driver's seat? What would your day be like if you had to find the way to the grocery store every time you left the house? Life would be catastrophically inconvenient! Our habits are not only biological but also have made modern life very easy. If we begin to harness them, we can use the power they have—not just passively, but consciously. This is the most crucial step to changing our lives for the better.

Our harmful habits are repetitive negative actions that can be changed to be repetitive positive actions. Here are everyday examples of energy expended in harmful habits that we have ingrained into our consciousness over time.

Examples of Harmful Habits

- Smoking
- Pacing
- Gambling
- Road Rage
- Fidgeting
- Lip or nail biting
- Overspending
- Procrastination
- Eating junk food
- Laziness
- Self-pity
- Cracking knuckles or joints

- Excessive grooming
- Overmedicating
- Self-harm behaviors
- Emotional abuse
- Judging other people
- Picking fights
- Talking over or ignoring others
- Neglect of grooming and hygiene
- Harassment and bullying
- Playing video games excessively
- Avoiding responsibilities
- Binge watching movies/TV shows
- Competitive feelings toward others
- Hate toward others
- Greed
- Breaking promises to yourself and other people
- Nervous talking
- Lying/spreading gossip or rumors
- Gut reactions like honking the car horn or yelling
- Excessive sexual activity
- Compulsive phone checking
- Internet/peer envy
- Constantly focusing on the negative
- Complaining without taking action to change your situation
- Drinking coffee, soda, or alcohol excessively
- Overeating
- Undereating or constantly dieting

- Picking (hair, skin, nails)
- Taking pills or doing drugs
- Overworking
- Excessive exercising

Harmful habits manifest in us for all kinds of reasons: to quell our nerves, to relieve our boredom, to escape from a life issue we don't want to face, or sometimes as a coping mechanism meant to "solve our problems." They're harmful because they're unconscious and usually uninhibited. Gone unchecked, they control us and can steer us far off course.

Most people don't really think about *why* they're really doing something. If you do, you're already ahead of the game. Most of us have our habits hardwired into us from our childhood or young adulthood. Often our habit is based on our past and is a way to cope with our fears about the future. With some practice, you'll start to recognize it easily: *Your harmful habit is a procrastination from your true purpose.* It halts your productivity and growth.

Let's work to identify some of your harmful habits. Take a minute and write down three harmful habits you have right now. Check the list above if you need a gentle reminder. We all engage in at least ONE of those harmful habits at one time or another. Be honest with yourself. Okay, got it? Now write them down:

Three of My Harmful Habits:

1. _____

2. _____

3. _____

Identifying your harmful habits gets easier over time. They will be your biggest distraction from your personal motivation and drive. For instance, you may want to get work done, but instead you smoke a cigarette or check an app. Or you may want to start a business and have more freedom, but instead you wake up at an ungodly hour to continue working for someone else at a job you hate. We all know this person: She desires to move to a place she really loves but instead sits around talking trash about her own town; he wants to paint, but instead he spends his afternoon making excuses for why he doesn't have the time and putting down the work of others.

These daily, mindless habits make and shape our lives, and getting a handle on what they are is the difference between a stagnant life and a productive one. Our habits *can* be what inspire us to get up extra early in the morning when they are *mindful,* but on most days, they are what encourages us to hit snooze and lounge around in bed. Often we don't even recognize that the "sleeping in" habit is harmful, but in the case of the snooze button, it's actually procrastination at it's finest. Procrastination is a way of obtaining instant gratification instead of focusing on the real goal of long-term success. That's why we need to learn not just how to recognize our habits, but how to transform them into positive, productive habits that propel us forward.

We can be destructive with our habits or we can learn to channel them and improve our lives. For instance, we can smoke every day, or we can begin the habit of replacing those cigarettes with a walk around the block or a mindful meditation. In my case, I took prescription pills every day for conditions I never should have been diagnosed with, but unfortunately the act of taking those pills became a habit. I learned how to replace that habit with one that was healthier for me: taking vitamins and minerals that truly support my health.

Think about some of your own life choices. Are your everyday activities supporting your health and growth in life or are they holding you back? Do they genuinely make you feel good about yourself—or are they things that cause you to feel guilty or that lower your self-esteem?

Explore the reasons you partake in the three harmful habits you recognized earlier. Again, be honest with yourself. We are now looking at ourselves without judgment, because this is the way to truly change. Facing your harmful habits may instantly reveal a new, helpful layer to your life. You may realize that you binge watch TV because it's been your "reward" since you were a kid, even though today you'd rather be spending quality time with your family. Write down the reason that each harmful habit is giving you an excuse. How is it holding you back? Your answers may help shed some insight on some of your habits.

Reasons for My Harmful Habits:

1. _____

2. _____

3. _____

Changing Your Habits

Most times we don't change because we want to change, we change because we *have* to change. Something external—such as a job loss, health scare, or divorce—forces us to change. As a matter of fact, all we usually need to convince us to make a major change is a glimpse into our future if we continue in our current direction.

I knew if I didn't make a change the very day I attempted suicide—strung out and at my absolute worst mentally—that I would never, *ever* make the change. I knew that if I waited to improve my habits and cut toxicity out of my life, I would be much worse off than I currently was, and my struggle would become much more difficult as time went on. For once, I gave different parts of my own psyche a front seat. I saw a glimpse of my future if I continued on my current path, and I did not like what I was seeing. In the end, if I was honest with myself, I knew in my heart that I was going to end up chronically ill or dead. Maybe you experienced a life event that woke you up and made you realize it was time to change your harmful habits, and that's why you've picked up this book. While a major life event can really motivate us to shift our perceptions, we don't have to hit rock bottom to get inspired to live a better life. We can still choose to take the time to truly think about our life and make the choice to change. Now.

How I did not die on fourteen prescription drugs—or coming off fourteen prescription drugs cold turkey!—is still a mystery to me and any medical professional who I've spoken to about my journey. I'll say this: In the midst of conquering horrendous withdrawal symptoms, I found a lot of clarity. Once I quit my job, I didn't give myself any other choice but to get well. I bought the cheapest blender I could find, invested in bulk bags of fruits, nuts, and vegetables for smoothies (the only thing my body could digest), and hunkered down in my apartment. For the first time ever, I could focus solely on the most important obligation of all: myself.

In the gaps between staring at the ceiling and leaning over into a garbage can, I had a lot of time to contemplate my life choices. Almost immediately, I began to see how my harmful habits had formed distinct, negative, and mostly unconscious patterns in my life that had led me to where I was: sick, sad, and in need of a major change.

I became inspired to improve my life, and with just a few tweaks in my day and in almost no time at all, I began to feel completely different—a way I had never even dreamed that I *could* feel. I was energized, inspired, and for once, I felt awake. I felt like I was seeing things through the eyes of a child. Everything was interesting and wonderful. Learning how to continue to improve became my life, and it was thrilling.

Soon enough, my entire life began to *look* completely different, exceeding my expectations at every turn. I attracted the kind of people who supported me. I learned who my true friends were. I purged negative people, toxic products, and unhealthy foods from my life. I started to recognize what "harmful" looked like in all its form, and I learned how to protect my own energy. I opened myself up to learning from others and met educators in functional medicine and gurus in meditation who guided and taught me. I was able to see myself as a part of the greater whole, which made me less focused on my own ego. I picked up books on Ayurveda and nutrition that truly healed me from ailments that had plagued me all my life. I began to recognize my body as a reflection of my true self: a vibrant and healthy person. Today I can happily say that I've saved my life, and through my work, many other people have told me that I've saved their lives, too. This is the most rewarding, incredible, satisfying part of all.

We all want to feel vibrant and balanced. Every one of us craves security and an enjoyable life. But often we unconsciously attract the wrong things or dwell in negative thoughts. What stops us from living our best lives? Often it's our habits—but we can change those habits to work to our advantage and lead us down a better path.

Choosing New WILD Habits

Here are some examples of new, WILD habits that can easily replace your harmful ones. We are all capable of doing at least one of the items on this list! Refer to the list whenever you're in a funk or need a quick idea to get you started. They're each fun in their own way and will help you on the way to a better life.

WILD Habit Examples:

Go for a walk.

Detox from your phone (try spending some time without your phone for the first hour of every morning, an hour before bed at night, and for the whole day on the weekends!).

Take vitamins and supplements that support your health *We'll cover many of these in chapters nine, ten, and eleven.*

Go to the beach.

Dance.

Sing.

Watch the sunset.

Get involved in a cause you love.

Spend time outside.

Write music.

Listen to music.

Participate in a retreat.

Say, "I love you; you're perfect" to yourself in the mirror.

Exercise.

Craft.

Create a blog.

Eat organic food.

Go for a hike.

Call a friend.

Create something with your hands.

Plant a garden.

Have an at-home spa day.

Talk to your family.

Practice meditation.

Paint.

Bring home a new plant.

Do an organic beauty ritual.

Take a bath.

Take a yoga class.

Cook your favorite colorful, organic meals.

Be kind to others.

Focus on your breath for five minutes.

Donate to a good cause.

Commit to a fitness plan.

Freewrite in your journal.
  Simply allow thoughts to come to you and write without crossing out or correcting anything.

Read a new book.
  Congrats, you're already doing this one!

Start a business.

Spend time with animals.

Express gratitude.

Write a book.

Start a charity.

You can even combine some of these new, WILD habits to see how wonderfully it affects you! For instance, you can take a bath while reading this book and free-writing in your journal. You can take a jog with your dog or a phone-free walk around the neighborhood with your sister. You can start a business that donates a percentage of its profits back to a cause you're passionate about. Now that we've identified some WILD habits, write down three that you're committed to practicing every day for the next month:

Three WILD Habits I Will Practice for Thirty Days:

1. _____

2. _____

3. _____

How will each WILD habit support you on the way to a better life? Maybe you're committed to spending more time with animals, so you start to take your dog out on a walk twice a day, or you stop to pet him for ten minutes instead of the usual two. That night he cuddles with you, which makes you feel intensely safe and happy. He's feeling your new bond. This new WILD habit has brought you joy. A study reported in the *Medical Journal of Australia* found that pet owners generally have lower blood pressure, triglycerides, and cholesterol levels than people who do not own pets.[1] Write down the three ways that these WILD habits will improve your life, either in the short or long term:

My WILD Habits Will Improve My Life by:

1. _____

2. _____

3. _____

Start By Loving Yourself

For the first couple of years after college, I worked day in and day out at a job I hated and then spent my precious time complaining about it. I lived in a city that made me feel unsafe, but I refused to move somewhere better. I dated people who were terrible for me, but I constantly craved their crazy brand of attention to validate my self-worth.

Nothing I did came from a pure, loving place, and furthermore, every time I acted out I reiterated to my body and my mind that this was the correct route to take with my feelings. I carved deep, dark neural pathways in my mind, and over time, I wondered why I was staring in the mirror at someone I didn't like at all.

I took pills that were causing bad effects on my body, but I thought I was doing the right thing because a doctor had diagnosed me, given me a prescription, and no other treatment options had been presented to me. The thing was, deep down, it never truly felt like the right thing. I *knew* somewhere inside myself that this was my harmful habit; I just didn't have a name for it at the time.

In attempting to make myself better, I realized that I had instead made myself much worse. The kinds of drugs I had put in my system every day for eleven years were only hurting me, especially when coupled together and layered on top of one another.

Addiction followed me outside of my family; almost everyone I dated was a completely different person while "under the influence." It seemed I was always stuck in relationships that were chaotic because unhealthy relationships were comfortable for me. My relationship with my mother was reflected in my relationships with just about everyone I dated: I was constantly caring for them, picking up after their messes, and crying that they didn't show up when I needed them.

While I always sang, wrote, painted, and read during my free time, I never felt that a career in any of these fields was viable. When a voice inside me had been loudly shaking me about what my future should be, I had sternly told that voice to shut up, sit down, and ignore my dearest creative dreams. *Now*, please.

My nutrition was poor, at best. I lived off of two hundred dollars a month in food stamps for many years, and I made it go as far as I could by buying cheap, poor cuts of meat, sugary foods, and soda. I doused everything with salt and never looked at ingredients or considered nutritional value. Since I had grown up using food stamps, and used them to pay for groceries well into my twenties, this practice seemed totally normal to me.

It's true what they say: You can't love another person unless you love yourself. Love must be directed within first, then shown outward toward others. Think of love like teaching—you can't teach a subject until you've mastered it. You can't give love unless you've mastered self-love.

I knew in my heart that the amount of medications I took were dangerous. Yes, perhaps more than one doctor had looked at my chart and somehow thought it was still A-OK to layer more meds on top of my regimen, but I had felt for years that it was harmful. I knew at twenty-one years old, when Ambien was making me black out, that these pills were detrimental, yet I continued to take them.

I continued to see doctors and allow them to prescribe me more pills on top of more pills. I never just flat-out refused. I never even got a second opinion for a single ailment I filled a prescription for. I never asked if there was another way. I never took my health into my own hands.

My choices had been terrible and harmful to my well-being. And when I could finally see my life without any judgment, when I could finally face my harmful habits with absolute clarity, I realized that for almost the entirety of my life I had failed to trust my own inner voice.

Find Your True Self

Galileo was imprisoned and punished for suggesting that the Earth was not the center of the solar system. He was right. But that means every other doctor and scientist of his time was wrong. I am here to remind you that every accepted scientific fact was once a harebrained theory, which then replaced a previously accepted scientific fact. People are wrong. They're subject to human error. Medicine and science are great, but they're called studies for a good reason. They are just that: an analysis done by man. They're limited to the confines of what can be observed.

I am not saying that we should not ever see a doctor or receive drugs or treatments. Of course, I believe in doctors and Western medicine. What I hope to point out is that many, many professionals have gotten it wrong over the years. Doctors are not divine; they're human. Science is not perfect; it's constantly evolving. It's just something to consider the next time you see a doctor or fill a prescription.

Doctors and scientists are people. They're responsible for some of the greatest achievements on earth, but they're not perfect. That's the beauty of human nature—there is no such thing as perfect. Perfect is not the goal. *Balance* is the goal, and when balance is achieved, a fulfilling life will follow naturally.

When balance was the goal, I channeled my creativity instead of stifling it. I examined my circumstances instead of dismissing them. And I overcame my fears instead of allowing my fears to imprison me.

My life was a reflection of my actions, and my actions were a reflection of what I believed about myself. No matter how much medication I took, I would always be unhealthy. No matter how much love I had, I would always feel lonely. No matter how much money was in my bank account, I would always be poor—that is, if I didn't change the way I *thought* and the way I cultivated my habits.

Life will have an effect on you. You may think you're "numbing out," but what you're really doing is missing out. Learning your daily tendencies and your most common habits and using them to better yourself is the only way to truly unlock your mind, channel your true self, and live your most authentic life.

Kristen's Story:
Change Your Habit, Change Your Life

Kristen stops at her favorite coffee shop every single morning before work. She drives by on her route, so it seems convenient enough. Each morning, she turns right into the parking lot, stops at the drive-through, orders her coffee, pays her $4.50, and then heads to work. She gets to indulge in her habit and she even receives a reward—her coffee buzz (and maybe even a friendly "hello" to the cute barista).

She's embarrassed about her car, though, and has been for a long time. Kristen has always driven a hunk of junk, and yet can't seem to save money for her dream car. She gets a daily reward while drinking her coffee, but her satisfaction only lasts a few short minutes while she sips her drink. Meanwhile, Kristen actually has plenty of coffee to drink at home. In fact, she could make a month's worth of coffee for about $5 if she took the time to brew her favorite brand, which she could easily buy at the grocery store.

Not only can Kristen save money by conquering her harmful habits but she can also open herself up to a completely new life. Say she cuts out her coffee shop stop from her route in the morning. This will improve her time management in multiple ways: Kristen doesn't have to get in her car to drive, she doesn't have to wait in line for her coffee or wonder how long the five cars in front of her will take to be served. It also improves her emotional experience. She doesn't expose herself to the morning anxiety of getting to work on someone else's timeline.

With one less stop to make on her way, Kristen doesn't feel as rushed. Her morning anxiety has melted away. She begins to enjoy a leisurely walk to work instead of her usual hurried drive. This in turn enhances Kristen's walking stamina, boosts her mood, and improves her cardiovascular health. On her way to work, she is still able to say her friendly "hello" to completely different, interesting people in a totally new way, leaving her open to fresh and exciting experiences and relationships every single day.

She starts making a warm tea to-go before she heads out to work, to keep her away from the coffee shop. It works! After some days at this new habit, Kristen's successfully avoided her harmful habit (and avoided her afternoon caffeine crash). Instead, she is naturally full of energy from her morning walk and green tea. She grabs a healthy salad at lunch, rather than a coffee refill.

Her new morning walking routine inspires Kristen to start running and going to the gym in her apartment building, activities that have incredible long-term health benefits, which she felt she "never had the time for" previously. Since Kristen is now saving on both coffee *and* car maintenance (gas, oil changes, and more), she's eventually able to afford a gently used version of the car of her dreams. In this way, she has become a healthier, wealthier, more balanced person and has accomplished many of her long-term goals, simply by switching *one* habit.

Conquering just one harmful habit and replacing it with a WILD habit can have positive consequences in dozens of areas of your life. Now we're going to learn how.

CHAPTER 3

The WILD Method

In the last chapter I helped you learn how to identify your harmful habits and gave you an idea of how to replace them with WILD habits. But why do I call them WILD habits and what exactly does that mean?

In this chapter I'll explain each step of the acronym and outline exactly how to follow the WILD Method when you are trying to replace your harmful habits with healthier ones. This method will keep you on the right track and remind you how to accomplish your goals, even when they seem impossible. I will show you how to apply the WILD Method to your life so that you can use it any time you are struggling to implement positive changes.

Nuture Your WILD Habits

Recasting your harmful habits into WILD habits is the first step to stopping your self-sabotaging behaviors. Self-sabotaging behaviors include thoughts and actions like:

- "I get it, but then because I don't believe I should have it, I blow it."
- "I want it, but I'll settle for less because I don't deserve it."
- "If I ignore or mask this problem, it will go away."
- "I want it, but deep down I feel like I don't deserve it."

- "If I get it, I'll feel guilty and depressed."

- "If I get it, I'll lose it."

- "If someone else has it, I want it."

- "I will never have it, so why bother?"

Self-sabotage is sneaky. It finds each of us at one time or another. That's why you need to form the tools to recognize it. If you do what it takes to bring your life into balance, you won't have regrets because your life will reflect exactly what you seek.

These tools will soon form your actions, which in turn will become your habits. The ancient Vedic text of Brihadaranyaka Upanishad, one of the oldest Upanishadic scriptures of Hinduism, says this about our actions:

> You are what your deep, driving desire is.
> As is your desire, so is your will.
> As is your will, so is your deed.
> As is your deed, so is your destiny.[2]

Our habits reveal our deepest desires. We may say we want to read a gossip column, but what we really want to do is escape our problems. By conquering a harmful habit, we can begin to recognize, face, and then solve our problems instead of running from them. By examining your habits, you begin to conquer your deepest desires, your intention, your will, your deed, and your destiny. Finding and cultivating our WILD habits is simple to remember. It lies in the term "WILD" itself:

> Willingness
> Intuition
> Love
> Discipline

Together, they form the WILD Method, a formula that you can easily use to tackle any habit for good. Using these four simple tools is precisely what you need to unlock your mind and unleash your true power.

Willingness

The "W" in WILD stands for willingness. This is not the same as willpower, which we build later. Willingness is about being prepared to do something differently. It's about being willing to acknowledge our harmful habits and want to take that initial first step toward a better life. It's this readiness to change that can truly tip the scale.

The first step to changing our lives is to be willing to see things differently. We have to surrender. In fact, finding our true selves lies in accepting that perhaps we haven't been seeing things right to begin with. Change doesn't just happen, not even when we want it to. We have to be prepared to change. *We have to be willing to change.*

I have a former colleague from Weill Cornell Medical Center, Justine, who was driven by a habit that's becoming more and more common these days—intense fixation. She could be (and often was) easily influenced by a single, curated social media account. Justine would sit on her phone for hours poring over one impossibly curvy girl's feed after the next. It seemed like she was totally fixated on wanting to look like a different airbrushed girl each week. Justine constantly talked about how much she envied the girls' bodies.

"Why can't I look like that?" she'd ask me, sighing.

"Do you think this is real or Photoshopped?" she'd inquire, shoving her phone an inch from my face.

"Her thighs . . . oh my god. Her thighs are GOALS, Tara! GOALS!" she'd say without even looking up at me once.

Before I knew it, Justine was texting me from a plastic surgeon's office, undergoing a risky, last-minute surgery that included breast augmentation, liposuction, and Botox injections.

"I went to his office on Monday and I just couldn't help myself!" she texted me.

It was Wednesday afternoon.

Believe it or not, many people are actually intensely driven by impure feelings, fueling habits that reflect jealousy and envy. These habits can be just as motivating (at least on a short-term basis) as love or ambition if you're in a negative mindset. With rampant internet envy on the rise, negative motivators are only becoming more and more ubiquitous. These habits are sometimes motivating, but as you'll come to see, they have no satisfactory ending for the person who experiences them.

After many weeks of recovery, Justine and I met for lunch at an organic cafe and I asked her how she felt after her surgery.

"Great!" she exclaimed.

I took a sip of my tea but before I could respond, she touched my hand. I looked up and into her eyes. Justine got quiet.

"Tara," she said to me, "I don't get it."

"Don't get what, love?" I asked. I had never seen this look in her eyes before. Justine looked panicked, almost desperate.

"I got the surgery, and I love my new boobs! You know I love them! Everyone knows I love them! Anyway, I got a new boyfriend—HE loves them! He's great. And my measurements are what I always wanted them to be! I know that I should be over the moon. I know I should be . . ."

"What's wrong?" I asked.

"I'm still not *happy*," she said, leaning in. "And I don't know why. It's like . . . nothing is *fixed*."

"Justi," I told her, meeting her eyes, "your body looks different, but you're right, in a way nothing *is* fixed. They did surgery on your body, not your brain. Your body is different, but your mind is *exactly the same*."

She broke down in tears then, covering her face and nodding over and over again into her hand. As I got up and hugged her, she confessed through sobs that even though her body was quite different, her *habits* had not changed at all.

Justine told me that every night she would sneak away from her boyfriend and go into the bathroom. During this time she would sometimes spend up to an hour engaging in the same behaviors as before. She would stare at girls and cry over why she did not look like them. She'd spend hours wishing that she had the body of someone else. She had changed things on the outside, sure, but on the inside, Justine confessed to me, she was still hurting a lot.

"My boyfriend thinks I'm taking a bath, but even in the bath, I just lean over and stare at my phone the whole time, hating myself. I hate myself," she told me. "I absolutely hate myself."

"No you don't," I told her. "Truly, you don't hate yourself."

I took her hand in mine and let her know the truth—the truth I had learned years before, at my most desperate place. I let her know the secret that had changed my life forever.

"Justine," I said, squeezing her fingers in my palm, "you don't hate yourself. You don't hate yourself in the least. You hate your habits. *You hate the fact that you sit around and hate yourself.* And that is your right. It's okay. You *should* hate that because I've seen it make you completely miserable. Hating that is the first step to changing it. You hate your habits, but you can change them. Your insides can match your outsides, and vice versa. You can fix this. You can be happy with who you are. It's NEVER too late. You'll see. I promise you: You don't hate yourself at all."

Justine's eyes lit up as she began to understand: It wasn't that she hated herself, it was that she hated the act of hating herself. She hated the *habit* of hating herself, which she had indulged in day after day for many years without thinking about the harm it was doing to her. It had negatively impacted her life in every way. Her harmful habits of comparison, competition, and intense fixation had led to impulsive decisions, superficial ego gratifications, and in the end held no happy ending. There would always be someone else there to envy. There would always be something else to be jealous of. She needed to change her habits or *nothing* was going to change. I wiped away her tears and I commiserated with her, because we've all been there: lost and distracted from our true purpose but finally ready—and willing—to change.

We identified that Justine's problem was intense fixation, or an extreme preoccupation with something or someone. This is a harmful habit that does not serve you, but that you engage in anyway, with a frequency of more than once a day. It often displays as a repetitive behavior, such as compulsive phone checking, internet stalking, drinking, popping pills, or nervous talking. This modern-day problem seems to affect a majority of the country. It shows up in a lot of ways and has received a lot of labels in the last century. We all know at least one person who displays the traits of this common habit.

On average, people in the United States across all age groups check their phones forty-six times per day, according to Deloitte. That's up from thirty-three looks per day in 2014. Collectively, Americans check their smartphones upwards of eight billion times *per day*. Informate CEO Will Hodgman said, "While social networking may have started as a viral craze for US teenagers, it's steadily matured into an everyday lifestyle for many adults around the world who are now eclipsing teens and young adults as most-frequent users."[3]

In a way, we've become addicted to watching other people's lives. We are consumers of each other. This habit can often lead to feelings of jealousy or envy. Habits built around jealousy, envy, and fixation never end in true success. True success is the knowledge deep down that you have contributed something of worth to the world.

Intense fixation habits leave us empty and they don't propel us to take productive, long-term action for ourselves or our future. They only fill short-term needs and keep us at a low mental and physical vibration (more on this later).

Justine's story is not unlike the realization many of us make. She had been willing to do everything to feel better—everything except the one thing she really *needed* to do. When in doubt, we need to look within to find the thing we need to change. But our ability to then change the habit of any repetitive thought or behavior is based on our *willingness.* Justine and I went through some of the questions outlined below, and she admitted to me that she had been willing to do the work on herself everywhere but on the inside. She spent her time fixated on others as a way to avoid having to face her real problems—the cause of her low self-esteem. She spent her time fixated on her body because she thought that changing her body would change her self-esteem. It was not until after plastic surgery that she realized that she still had to put in the work for self-love: Nothing else was going to create self-love for her.

Three Questions to Invoke Your WILLINGNESS to Change

1. Am I satisfied with my current circumstances?

2. What would I like my life to look like?

3. What am I willing to do to have that life?

Be sure to come back to these questions every few weeks and see how your answers grow and change. As you take steps to change, the answers to these questions will change. When you avoid your problems, you avoid your personal growth. You can tackle this by asking yourself what you are fixing and what you are ignoring. To see a shift in your life, be willing to switch things up: If you're not satisfied with how much money you have in your bank account, you can find a good mentor on money management (someone you know who has been successful) and ring them up for advice. You can begin saving and putting a certain percentage of every paycheck in the bank. With this new WILD money habit, you can live an easier lifestyle where money is no longer a stress for you. You can even set yourself up for a life where money is no object.

Create goals that fulfill your deepest desires. There is a small, powerful way to accomplish your deepest desires, and it's worked for me and countless others. Begin a journal where you write down your goals on one page. You may start here and then transfer it over to a journal, if it helps you to begin right now.

My Goals

1. _____

2. _____

3. _____

4. _____

5. _____

Read this list every night before you go to bed and consciously imagine yourself accomplishing each goal as you go down your list. Mentally picture each and every step it would take to accomplish each goal. Repeat this exercise every night and again in the morning if you so choose. It may take you less than five minutes, but as you'll see, it's incredibly powerful. You'll be pleasantly surprised by

how many seemingly impossible goals become possible the moment
you begin to picture them really happening!

As you begin to accomplish these goals in real life, simply check
them off. Add on new goals if you like, but continue to read your
list every night until each goal is accomplished. (Don't worry, we'll
outline many of the steps that make your goals achievable in the
coming chapters, so you'll know just what to do!) Once you start
asking yourself questions and creating intentions that focus on self-
improvement, it will be easier to recognize the patterns that have
been holding you back. When you can recognize these distinct patterns, you can begin to invoke your willingness to picture your life
in a brand-new light. You'll be able to start fresh. An open mind can
lead to a vastly improved existence.

Intuition

Intuition is where the "I" of the WILD Method comes in. Your
intuition lies in your ability to perceive your world accurately—to
observe your reality and match it up to your expectations. To con-
front your perceived unworthiness and your real issues head on,
without excuses, is an important part of this. Your intuition truly
rests in your ability to separate opinions from facts. Once you trust
your intuition and use it to your advantage, you're well on your way
to a more manageable, happier life.

The more we use our intuition, the easier it becomes to see ourselves clearly and honestly. After invoking our willingness to change
and taking a good honest look at our faults (without judgment!), we
need to use our personal intuition to conquer our habits. After all,
we know ourselves best. Calling on your personal intuition provides
you with the real insight into what you need to do in order to change
your life and how to actually move forward. This is where most
people fall short. There is little sense in being willing to change if

we don't trust our intuition and act on it. Acting on your intuition moves you closer to your goal.

It's not enough to figure out our harmful habits. Identifying our harmful habits is not the same as addressing them or turning them into WILD habits. One of the first exercises I used with Justine was to have her use her intuition to find the *core need* of her habit. The core need is the "why." In Justine's case, it was *why am I fixated on other women's bodies?*

Ask yourself these questions to tune into your intuition and find the core need of your harmful habit:

My Core Needs

1. Why am I doing it?

2. What feeling am I after?

3. What need am I trying to fulfill?

Our intuition is the insight we have into ourselves as well as the world. It's our immediate apprehension—our direct perception of truth. Our intuition will easily tell us our "why." On the surface, Justine's "why" was insecurity. She fixated on other women's bodies because she felt deep down that she deserved to feel inferior. To fulfill her need to compare herself to others, she acted out in the form of putting herself down. Fixation and comparison may be meant to motivate us to improve, but instead of driving us to get better, they actually become incredibly destructive and damaging to us. Comparison puts the focus on the wrong person. When we constantly compare ourselves to others, we waste precious energy focusing on other people's lives rather than keeping our focus on improving our own life. Comparisons often result in envy and feelings that life is unfair. We never really know as much as we think we do about other people's lives, and furthermore, there is really no end to this harmful habit, no matter how successful we become. There will always be someone or something else there to steal your focus.

While the internet and social media can be inspiring and a little envy is probably harmless, engaging in acts of comparison is unhealthy and unproductive for us. Comparison robs us of our joy. Researchers surveyed nearly five hundred teens and found that those with lower self-esteem reported greater vulnerability to jealousy and aggression. A 2017 survey of more than five thousand American teens found that three out of four owned an iPhone. Jean Twenge, a professor at San Diego State, argues that smartphones may be destroying a generation of teenagers. "The more time they spend looking at screens, the more depressed they say they feel—there's not a single exception among any age group," Twenge says.[4]

Effects only get worse the longer we engage in a harmful habit. If we don't gain an awareness of this bad behavior in our adolescence, we can carry it with us throughout our whole life.

On a deeper level, our real "why" is often that we want something to motivate us to have control. We want the control it would take to improve our life. We want a supportive role model to inspire us to become the best version of ourselves. We want a reason to get better, fitter, and be able to look in the mirror with a smile on our face.

Justine wanted control and improvement, but instead she was getting disorder and disappointment. Trying to control her life by comparing herself to others was not the answer. It would never work. Comparison and fixation were bound to bring on more of the same destructive feelings that had brought Justine so much unhappiness to begin with, resulting in an endless loop of self-defeat. It wasn't a satisfactory form of control because it didn't rely on the most important person of all: herself.

You can only control one life and that's yours.

Love

Love may be the most important step in the WILD Method. Without it, the rest easily crumbles. If you do everything with love, you win. There is not a time that you'll feel judgmental, you won't cloud yourself with envy, and you won't waste your time with hate. You'll have no desire to procrastinate. You'll instantly be able to control how much you eat. Greed will disappear. Water the seeds of what you want to become with love. Practice love the same way you'd practice any discipline: with intense repetition. WILD habits require practice. When it's hard to love, that's when you know you have to practice love the most. Practice love. Repeat love.

Look within and determine your main passion. Search your mind for a hobby that you love or really miss. Some people love to write, dance, sing, solve math problems, paint, knit, read, build, nurture others, play golf, swim, run, or practice yoga. However, our self-sabotaging behaviors get in the way of these natural tendencies toward self-loving actions and often inhibit us from achieving or feeling true success. You'll recognize these behaviors when you see them—they're the most obnoxious forms of procrastination like gossip, judgment, negative thinking, self-loathing, and self-sabotage. And these behaviors can become habits, too. Constant negative thinking or self-loathing keeps us paralyzed and unable to embrace our true passions. Sometimes our mental and emotional habits can be the most harmful of all. We cannot ignore the power of our mind and its potential effect on our life path, as we'll see in the next chapter.

Instead of dwelling on what you don't have, *focus on what you want*. Whatever it is you want, keep your focus on it. People very rarely accomplish something the very first time that they go after it. You need to practice in order to see results. Whatever you want, practice having it. If you want to be a great singer, you practice. You sign up for vocal lessons. You learn songs that push your range. You learn how to read music. You live, eat, and breathe music. You love singing and you love hearing yourself sing. That's when other people love hearing you sing, too, and your passion can become your livelihood.

You can practice love in this same way. Whatever you want to do in life, start taking the self-loving steps to get there and make your goal attainable. Practice love no matter what another person's reaction is. Practice love no matter how disappointing life seems. No matter how difficult or insurmountable your circumstances may be, always show love. Practice love by first giving yourself a fighting chance to do and to possess the things you truly love.

The New Habit

I asked Justine what new habit she could easily replace her harmful habit with that would actually give her the benefits she was searching for: motivation, self-improvement, and constant inspiration. After a few minutes, Justine laughed.

"Reading," she told me, almost sheepishly. "I really like sitting somewhere and reading, but I haven't read a book in ages. I used to love reading, but now I'm too busy staring at this thing." She waved her cell phone around with a knowing smile and continued, "Being on my phone is like reading. Scrolling is like reading. But it's not really the same, is it?"

"Not at all," I said. We both laughed. "But what a relief! Reading is great for you and there is hardly anything better for inspiration, motivation, and the drive to self-improve than a good book. Let's get you reading the right things!"

After we wrapped up our lunch, I took Justine to the nearest library, just a few blocks away. As we entered the building, I noticed she was glowing. A big smile appeared on her face.

"I love the smell in here," she said, taking a deep breath. "Smells like being a kid."

When we checked out, Justine had five books in her hand: *Bossypants* by Tina Fey, *The Girl with the Lower Back Tattoo* by Amy Schumer, *#GIRLBOSS* by Sophia Amoruso, *The Diary of Anne Frank*, and *The Alchemist* by Paulo Coelho. I also gifted her my first self-help book, *Cured by Nature*.

She was on her way.

Today, Justine has changed her habit of scrolling through her phone to reading books that inspire her. She still sits in the bath every single night, but now, she reads the books and stories of her personal heroes. She has found her supportive role models: They are the heroes and heroines in the pages of her favorite novels. They are the authors who write the pages she's so often engulfed in. In books, Justine has found her source of self-improvement and motivation. Justine still uses social media, but she has worked on doing it consciously instead of unconsciously.

This has all been a vivid expression of self-love. She now uses that same intense fixation that used to make her miserable to run a successful beauty business of her own. Justine is still high-energy, but today she has an inner glow that people always comment on. She loves her job bringing healthy cosmetics to the market and is one of the happiest, most outgoing women I know. She is also one of the smartest and wittiest. Justine's knowledge of the world and her insight into herself and others is admirable—ever since she picked up the habit of reading every single night.

Self-love is another way of expressing self-compassion. For instance, you may get angry frequently toward people you love, then feel disappointed in yourself for losing your temper. Or you may be prone to self-doubt, which manifests as an anger or rash behavior toward yourself and others. It may seem like you have no control of your emotions, or that your temper has complete authority over you. However, without love and compassion for yourself, you are giving your negative mental and emotional habits all of the power instead of allowing your natural tendencies to guide you to your best life.

Anger is a form of passion, but this emotional habit steals our rationale and our problem-solving capabilities. We lose our ability to change the situation by being so negatively affected by it. Wrath does not change the world—compassion and understanding do. Forgiving yourself and having empathy toward yourself is the ultimate method of self-love. This is a crucial step to taming our harmful habit, because love will radiate from you and positively affect everyone you meet, and it will help you to see that you are worth changing. You can begin to bring love, care, and grace into everything you do. People will be more prone to listen to you. You will find that when you are kinder to others, they become kinder to you. Wrapped in love, anger naturally melts away.

Whether your harmful emotional habit is anger, guilt, self-loathing, or something else, learning to love yourself is the key to breaking any of these habits. Love is also an important part of the WILD Method because when you want to break a harmful habit, you not only need the willingness and intuition to do so but also the self-love to forgive yourself and proceed on a healthier path. When you truly love yourself, you have the self-worth to believe in yourself and remain focused on your WILD habits.

Love can also play a crucial role in replacing negative physical habits with WILD habits. Think back to those passions and hobbies that you enjoy. When you've reached the point where your intuition is telling you to change, and you are finally willing, those activities that you love can become your new WILD habits. Many times we are looking to satisfy a deeper emotional craving, not a physical one.

For example, if your harmful habit is comforting yourself with junk food and you know it's having a detrimental effect on your health, try replacing it with another activity that you love. Instead of reaching for that bag of chips, reach for your paintbrush, knitting needles, or journal.

Here are three questions to start taking self-loving action, especially when it's the most difficult:

1. What brings me joy?

2. How can I bring that joy into my life every day?

3. How can the things that make me happy make others happy, too?

Discipline

This is where the last step in the WILD Method becomes momentous: Discipline. With discipline, you can change these unconscious reactions instantly. When you do, you'll begin to see massive improvements in your own life right away. Discipline is what drives you to follow through with changing your harmful habits into WILD habits.

The grass isn't greener on the other side—it's greener where you water it. When you act with pure grit, discipline, and sheer determination, you are reinforcing your other positive steps: willingness, intuition, and love. This solidifies the positive path both literally (to the neurons in your brain) and figuratively (to the actions in your life).

The more you practice discipline in your positive habits and ideals, the more grooves you wear in this mental maze and life path. The more you wear this path, the easier this habit becomes. Nutritionists often advise their clients to follow a diet for thirty days because it will become a new habit and their brains will be rewired to want to continue this healthier path. It's the same with implementing your WILD habits—the more time you can commit to these new actions, the more ingrained they will become. Soon, it will be second nature to trust yourself and listen to your gut. Your intuition will grow stronger and synchronicities will manifest for you. Miracles will show up for you, people will find you just when you need them, and circumstances will align all around you.

Before she picks up her phone, Justine now asks herself just one simple question: *Why?*

She continues to ask herself *Why* until she gets to the root of her impulse. "If the answer is anything other than an emergency, a loved one, or an urgent work task, I pick up a book or go for a walk instead," she tells me.

I can tell that she no longer regrets her cosmetic choices, and she has chosen a path that provides nontoxic options to women as a way to give back. Justine promotes health and is an exemplary role model for the wellness community. Instead of spending hours wishing she looked like other women, Justine spends every waking hour making sure other women don't have to spend a moment feeling ugly. She turned her harmful habit into a successful business, and I've been so proud to watch it grow. This has all been a conscious expression of Justine's Willingness, Intuition, self-Love, and most importantly her Discipline to stay the course.

Every decision you make is a choice between getting better or getting worse: There is no standing still. You'll begin to have automatic, positive mental habits through increased Discipline, and all the other steps in the WILD Method—Willingness, Intuition, and Love—will also increase and expand. The more you reinforce an action, the more easily you can accomplish it the next time.

For instance, maybe you find yourself on a shopping app every night, even though it gives you a headache every morning when your bank account is negative again. Your "why" for your shopping habit is that you want the satisfaction. You crave the excitement of something new, but you know that your "shopping hangover" is real. You don't really have money for bills or organic food or good lifestyle changes because you feel like you absolutely NEED the newest pair of shoes.

We don't really shop to shop. We shop to fulfill a need: a sense of euphoria, social acceptance, or a feeling of intoxication at getting a new item, for instance. But it fades every time—and almost instantly. Having a new shirt feels great in the moment, but when you've worn it for a month and it's made a cameo on social media, the "new shirt" feeling wears off. And really, our needs are never met. We don't ever get the satisfaction that we're truly after in the long term. Find your "why" and fulfill your need while cutting out your harmful habit.

You can replace the habit of shopping with the habit of donating. Any time you feel that you have some extra money to spend on yourself, ask yourself if you're spending that money wisely. It's okay to be self-indulgent every once in a while, or to buy a new outfit for a certain event or special occasion, but before you spend your hard-earned money on frivolous things that are self-serving, do a bit of research to see who might be in need right now.

With this small switch, you are upgrading your "me" mentality to an "us" mentality. You have started to include other people in your fortune. You've begun to search for people in need, putting yourself in a greater position to serve. Instead of spending fifty dollars on yourself, you may find a different charity to give a dollar to for twenty days, and put the rest away in a savings account. It feels so great to give, because you meet giving people and begin to feel gratitude for what you have. It feels wonderful to save because it makes you far less stressed out. It will make you feel so good it will be easy to keep up your discipline in this WILD habit.

Through this new WILD habit, you finally receive the long-term satisfaction that you've truly been seeking. Instead of doing this once, you start to do this every single night for a month. You like it so much (because it works!) that you decide to increase your new ritual to three months. If you can remain disciplined for a few weeks, this will become your new WILD habit. You'll become more knowledgeable about the world. You'll help others in a real and important way. You'll become more selfless. You'll experience the benefits that an education in humanity_has to offer you to solve your problems. You won't suffer from your morning "shopping hangover," you won't suffer from the ill effects of selfishness, and you won't find yourself focusing on your wants quite as often, because you will be too busy focusing on the world's needs. A healthier, happier you can emerge sooner than you'd ever imagine.

What you focus on will grow. Happiness and a great life are reflections of your habits. A positive mental habit can be planted, sewn, and cultivated over time. With discipline, you can harvest your own happiness intentionally and on a long-term basis.

After implementing Willingness, Intuition, and Love, intense Discipline will be easier to recognize and stick to by asking yourself these questions:

1. How has my behavior changed?

2. How has this positively affected my life?

3. How will I follow through on my goals today?

Applying the WILD Method

I truly did not know if, when, or how my withdrawals would end. I never knew anyone who had come off a major pharmaceutical medication, and I had been told my entire life not to quit my meds.

I had seen my mom detox from heroin at home, alone. No doctors and no drugs—this was ten times worse.

Doctors had told me since I was thirteen that coming off my meds was not an option because it was dangerous, unpredictable, and could kill me. They were right, I will say that much. I could have easily died, either from dehydration, weight loss, nutritional deficiency, putting stress on my organs, falling, or simply throwing up while I was asleep. Any of these things could have strained my body so much that it just gave up. My frame has always been tiny, and I really didn't have a pound to lose.

I'm no different from anyone else. I'm not particularly gifted with immense willpower. I had never quit anything before in my life. Without the WILD Method, I would have given in many times—if nothing else, to stop the withdrawals. My body was so addicted to these drugs, and I hadn't even realized it! People ask me now how I've remained free from medications for seven years and not turned back to some of the most addictive drugs known to man. I took fentanyl for two years. Without the WILD Method, I'm not sure how I would have stayed off it all this time.

I didn't give in because I had the **willingness** to acquire the inspiration to change my life for the better. I didn't relapse because I had the **intuition** to see why I was making this choice. I didn't give up because I **loved** myself enough to remind myself that withdrawals were temporary but good health was permanent. I didn't give up because of my persistent **discipline** to my task of achieving wellness. The discipline I had to continue this cycle of healthy choices was the only reason I kept on, even when every single bone in my body was screaming at me to give in and give up. No one had told me to come off my drugs, so no one would have faulted me for going back on them.

These four simple steps are what kept me away from the orange bottles for the first few weeks. These steps are what led me to take a garbage bag full of pills (all the Rx meds I'd been prescribed, many of which hadn't worked) and twist the top. The WILD Method is what enabled me to bring that bag of pills to the curb and never look back.

Ever since making this shift, I've approached everything in my life in exactly the same way. Using the WILD Method, I've also been able to help others figure out their harmful habits and find a new path to a happy, successful, stable life. It has been one of the most rewarding parts of this journey. It was something I used to dream of that is now very much real.

⌘⌘⌘⌘

Would it surprise you to learn that much of the dissatisfaction in your life is reinforced for you, day in and day out, purely out of habit? It's true. Master your habits, and you can master your entire life. You now have all the steps necessary through the WILD Method. They can be applied to any area of your life.

We are at the center of many unexplored mysteries, all of which can change us. Incorporating WILD daily rituals that eventually replace your harmful habits will help you to do everything from quieting your mind to fueling your body. Through the WILD Method, you can find your bliss, recognize the wisdom that's in nature, and attain self-mastery. Life can be profoundly inspiring, extraordinary, and miraculous. You can take back your health, unleash your mind, and unlock your true power.

Don't just survive in this marvelous, mysterious universe—thrive in it!

CHAPTER 4

Committing to the WILD Method

You can take anything from Valium to Xanax to herbal teas, but if you're not in the right state of mind, it's not going to change much. Everyone has down days. Everyone has days when feeling better seems impossible. Even people who you consider to be permanently cheery have moments of despair and sadness. This is totally normal. It's okay. It's healthy. Feeling is dealing.

However, prolonged sadness or allowing terrible feelings to take over days or weeks of your time is not only no fun but also a habit that gets more and more difficult to pull yourself out of the longer it victimizes you. I've felt the desperate feelings. I've had the ugly cry. I've drowned in the insecurities. I've let myself feel all the emotions and have typical (and sometimes atypical) breakdowns. But now after I've let it all out I'm able to take inventory of my emotions in just a few minutes and take myself back to center. I can take a moment, disconnect from the intense negativity, and allow myself to indulge in feelings of absolute happiness.

The tools in this book have worked for me in the years I've been practicing them and for many others for thousands of years. Today, I've been off my medication for over half the time I was on it. I can say with absolute clarity that I never needed it to begin with. I've accepted that without judgment or anger or resentment. It just is, and as long as I do better every single time in the future, it all had a purpose.

The beauty of acceptance and allowing yourself to feel however you're feeling in the moment will bless you with the clarity of clear perspective. So it's okay if you're struggling to change your harmful habits into improved, WILD habits. You may encounter some setbacks. Change is hard, but if you call upon your *Willingness, Intuition, Love,* and *Discipline* then I know you can do it.

No matter where we're at in life, there is almost always something, however small, that is blocking our way. That "thing" normally stems from a fear. A fear of the unknown, a fear of failure, or even a fear of success! Sometimes it comes in the form of resentment, stress, anxiety, or sadness. Many of us recognize that we often manifest our fears, but we still don't know how to stop them.

Goal setting is great. But goal accomplishing? Well, that's the best feeling in the world. It's having your dreams turn into reality before your very eyes. Goal setting and accomplishing is what's gotten me from New York to California, has taken me from strung-out pillhead to sober life-a-holic and has sailed me from anxiety-ridden damsel to completely kick-ass and happy boss babe CEO.

Goal accomplishing has done more good for my life and made me feel better than any material thing, any person, any situation, or any drug. It's shaped my life more than any exercise or any experience. Accomplishing your goals is the ultimate drug if you do it right. In this chapter I will show you exactly how to achieve your goals and WILD habits by changing the way you think, maturely dealing with your setbacks, and finding freedom in following through with your purpose.

Freedom From Judgments

True freedom. What is it, anyway? Is it found in a ballot box? At the top of a mountain? Miles out to sea? Or is it found in the soul, in your choices, and in your actions?

Bullies used to throw my lunch away and trip me in hallways during high school. The young ladies that I went to academy with used to love teasing me mercilessly. Now they like my Instagram photos and congratulate me on Facebook. They ask me for health and beauty advice.

It doesn't really matter what we choose to do in life—whether you spend your life on a couch or jet setting around the world—someone is going to judge you for it. Judgment is completely universal. Yes, even the most pious, sexy, or admirable people (take Gandhi, Marilyn Monroe, and JFK, for example) were all judged in their lifetimes and continue to be long after.

I mean, even Jesus had haters. Consider it a rite of passage into the real world.

I used to be ruled by my relationships. Not just my relationships with my significant other, either. I cared a tremendous amount about what my friends, teachers, family, mentors, and even (or especially?!) strangers thought of me. Strangers! I mean, how silly is that?

It took a lot of reading, meditation, and soul-searching, but unless I really, truly care about someone, most people's observations about what I'm capable of or who I truly am can just disappear. I'm totally up for hearing people's opinions, and often even use them as insight or apply them to my life. But judgments, rumors, and theories from other people don't even go in one ear to make it out the other. They simply don't exist. So don't listen when others tell you that you can't change your harmful habits into WILD ones. You can.

Criticism and negativity are really just someone else's point of view. We're all entitled to these viewpoints, and we are also entitled to be completely wrong. Should you care what others think of you? No. Is this incredibly hard, especially when it's the opinion of a mentor, parent, sibling, teacher, or significant other? Of course.

But caring about the negative opinions of others is a distraction from your true purpose.

I'm sure you've heard the phrase, "You're the average of the five people you spend the most time with." It's a sentence first coined by Jim Rohn, one of my dearest mentors. Stay stuck in harmful habits, and it's a near guarantee that your circle of influence—your friends and your circumstances—will reflect those same unhealthy patterns, too. Sometimes the people around you are loving and supportive. Sometimes they're depressed and miserable. You can bet that whoever you keep for company is a current reflection of the habits you're exhibiting. Maybe not everyone, but certainly the five people you spend the most time with. Improve your habits using the WILD Method and you'll attract great company; the kind of people who are kind, nurturing, and understanding. Practice your WILD habits, and you'll attract the kind of people who will support them.

I've never received negative criticism from anyone I admire or trust. In fact, all of the people I really look up to understand and adopt wholeheartedly what's called *constructive criticism,* which is a method of expressing one's opinion that's designed to help the other person do better by offering helpful solutions. The people who are the harshest critics are creative cowards who risk absolutely nothing and invent very little. It's easy for lazy people to point out what you're doing wrong, but is it really that helpful to give them all the power? You know it's not, so take your power back!

The truth is, most criticism is irrelevant. The act of harping on negative thoughts has no place in success stories. Adapt to pick up on the vibes around you and then learn from them. This is part of using your intuition. If you know a situation is going to be toxic, don't enter into it. Learn how to empower yourself instead of focusing on fitting into what others say they expect from you. Maybe now is not the right time to ask your boss for a raise. Maybe this week it's a bad idea to bring your problems to a friend. Maybe you should skip that party this weekend. You can learn to diffuse the situation, but you also have a really beautiful option: Walk away. For instance, you may speak with someone who puts you in a negative mood for a moment, but that doesn't have to put you in a bad mood for the next day or the next week! This is your experience and yours completely. Life rarely hands us opportunities like that, so make the most of it and make it empowering. Think of the good times, laugh through the bad times, forgive yourself, let yourself have some inspiring aha moments, and then relax. There is nothing more you could have done or said.

Walk away from the people around you who aren't doing well for themselves. Some people are angry at life. Some people blame everyone else for their problems. Some people think everyone is out to get them. Some people think the world is rotten and they're destined to be broke or sad. Some people just simply don't want to ever get better. Getting to know what toxic looks like to you and how it's affected you throughout your life is crucial. This can be a huge life (and time) saver. You don't want to get stuck with people who will encourage your harmful habits and derail your WILD ones.

Trying to change people will surely help you realize how silly it is, and you'll instantly find way more productive things to do, such as focusing on your own goals or helping other people. If I caught myself judging, I instantly indulged in my WILD habits instead of my harmful ones. If I had a judgment about someone else or I caught myself about to partake in a harmful habit, I immediately switched gears. I got up (isn't it weird how you're often sitting when you engage in these things? Stagnation is the trigger for many harmful habits), I changed my posture, I edited some photos, I started my daily gratitude list. I worked on an article for my blog, or I reached out to an organization I loved, or I checked out what Oprah was up to on Instagram. I got myself off the negative thought I was on and onto a thought that propelled my life forward. I recognized that if I was doing anything other than bringing joy into my life, I was wasting my time. Everyone is doing the best that they can do at any given time. If you understand this, you can easily practice reserving your opinions of others. Slowly, your feelings about judgment will adjust.

When I indulged in my new WILD habits, I attracted the kind of people who really understood what I needed. My new friends are amazing, and with social media, the web of incredible souls that I connect with expands every day. I've found myself engaged with the right type of people, who really understand me and get my vibe, who understand my dreams and my limits, who teach me to dive deeper and to accept love and support. We've been able to help each other grow, because we are here to propel each other's goals in life. If my friends succeed, I succeed. If people in my community succeed, I succeed. We are always there for one another, without ever having to ask for favors. Friends reach out just when I need to hear from them. People arrive in my life just when it makes sense to meet them. After so many years of feeling like I never fit in anywhere, I've finally found my tribe.

When I see the tendency in other people to put away their life goals and dreams for someone or something else, I just want to shake them and scream, "Noooo!" Your mother, lover, brother, sister, friends, and employers don't determine what you're worth. You do. You WILL find other people who love what you love and understand what you need. You only need to embody those things, and similar people will be attracted to your energy. If you project love, they will give love. A positive mindset and a negative life are incompatible. They cannot exist simultaneously. If you are positive, loving, and engaging in activities that make you happy, that is precisely what your entire life will reflect.

On average, Americans have approximately three to five careers in a lifetime (for real, I have three to five careers right now!). Why? Because we're constantly evaluating and reevaluating what we're good at, and we crave change. And hopefully, we feel that we're worth more than what we were worth yesterday, or even a few moments ago.

You're not the same person you were a decade or even a day ago. You don't have the same body, and your cells have literally regenerated so many times that the original, infant and child you no longer exists in any way, shape, or form in this current moment. Embrace that. It's awesome.

If you want your life to look different—if you want to see the world, or start running, or lose weight, or quit your job—I only know one way to get there: Do it. Putting the blame on others for your faults or giving yourself excuses not to live the life you want is depriving yourself of what you know you truly deserve. Your family, your teachers, your friends, and people who don't even know you at all will admire and respect you. More importantly, *you* will respect yourself. Whatever, whomever you want to be, put it out into the world without shame.

If you do this, people around you will follow suit. Like attracts like. Try it and see!

Avoid Toxic People

Never forget that when someone judges you, it isn't in any way about you at all. It's about them and their own insecurities, needs, and limitations. People who are the most difficult to please are almost always the very people who are the least worth pleasing. They're the same people that will never be happy no matter what you do, because happiness is not on their radar. They create very little. Because they are focused solely on being the victim, they rarely give themselves a chance to bring anything of worth into the world.

When you are at happy and at peace, you feel no need to spread negativity. You can't focus on greed. You can't thrive on envy. You don't care what happened five years or even five seconds ago. When you're genuinely happy, doing things you truly love, there is no room for negative thoughts or hateful feelings towards others. When you are struggling, you judge. When you are not struggling, life is positive.

Toxicity is different. It's easy to recognize, but may seem difficult to stop. It's the people in our lives who are often the largest difference makers, but their harmful habits can often influence our own. A spark of romance can be our greatest inspiration. An unhealthy relationship can be our largest excuse. Don't wait to take this situation seriously. Just like any toxic food or poison, these negative, destructive people are extremely dangerous. They distract us from our positive or productive WILD habits. They'll be the people discouraging you from exercise or making fun of you for wanting to be a better person. They'll come up with reasons for you to stay in other bad relationships. They'll be the ones encouraging you to accompany them to the drive-thru for fast-food. Toxic people get you stuck in the past and focused on the negative, and in that mentality you can't move forward and you can't succeed. It is impossible for them to share in your joy.

Emotionally impaired people can try to cling onto you—sometimes for years! They can make you feel guilty, and because of that are not always easy to remove from your life. To help you detox your relationships once and for all, begin by using the WILD method.

The first step to getting rid of something—or someone—with a seriously negative influence on you is being *willing* to recognize the fact that this is harming you. Toxic people are manipulative and often extremely self-centered. They're difficult to please and draining to be around. They have a very difficult time owning their feelings or apologizing to you, and they will consistently make you prove yourself to them. They may even have spent so much time forcing you to focus on them, that you never had any time to take a step back and realize what a horrible impact that they've had on your life!

Use the WILD Method to Rid Toxicity in Your Life:

- ∾ Be *Willing* to recognize that you're dealing with a toxic person. Accept that based on previous experience, your brain has given you a warning sign that tells you when something or someone may harm you. This is your time to listen to that warning.

- ∾ Use your *Intuition* to ask yourself: *How does this person make me feel? What energy do they have? What are they focused on?*

- ∾ *Love* yourself enough to walk away when you're facing someone toxic. Set boundaries for yourself that you won't pass, such as "I will only text this family member instead of talking to them on the phone" or "I won't unblock them from social media."

- ∾ Stay *Disciplined* in the positive actions you take to remove them from your life. Stick to the boundaries you've set— no matter what! Do not change your mind six days or six months from now. Once you've made the decision to rid yourself of a negative person, stand firm in that decision.

If this person shows major changes over the course of many months, that's one thing. But remember that your *discipline* is about staying focused on what's best for you, not what's best for them.

If you're meant to be in one another's lives, eventually you will be. Sometimes that takes a lot of personal growth on both sides.

Overall, it's best to set boundaries and stick to them. Enforce your boundaries constantly or toxic people will use absolutely any weakness in your conviction over time to sneak back into your life. Energy flows where attention goes. The more selective you are about where your focus is, the more successful you'll be. The more time you spend away from toxic people and their harmful habits, the more time you have for yourself and the people who are positive, uplifting, and important to you. Make time for people who bring you happiness, and let go of those who bring you anything less.

Master the Follow-Through

Those who fail are easily influenced and swayed by the opinions of others. Opinions are the cheapest commodities on earth: Everyone has one. Reach your own decisions and follow through with them, even if others are being discouraging. Try not to let others derail you from your WILD habits. Stay the course and remain committed to your goals.

In sports, a good follow-through maintains a flow in the motion. It is to hit "smooth," rather than to hit "hard." It maintains a certain looseness in the swing, rather than tension or over-hitting the ball with too much power. Golf works in this way. If you don't follow through with your shot, you'll find yourself constantly missing your mark. Interestingly enough, scientists have explained that it's NOT exactly the follow-through that makes your shot go in smoothly and with precision. In fact, they've proven that simply *setting your mind up to follow through* gives you a much higher success rate. Just planning your follow-through can set up the end points of a trajectory that enables you to hit the ball with the maximum amount of force and control at the point of impact. This same theory applies to creating new WILD habits.

You may try something for a week or two, but that doesn't make it a new habit. That's why when we practice a workout routine for a short period of time, it doesn't stay with us forever. It is the act of sticking with something, even against all odds, that makes an impact on our lives. It's our persistence and determination—our *discipline*—that allows us to not only know something intellectually, but also to follow through and master it. When we've mastered a new habit, it becomes automatic. Our reactions are peaceful, miracles show up for us, and we expect and receive goodness from others— no matter what.

The most successful people have one habit in common: They reach decisions quickly, easily, and they rarely change their minds. This is most likely why managers and CEOs have reputations for being stubborn. It's not by accident. They've cultivated a habit of *knowing what they want*, and often they refuse to compromise. This may be viewed as "bossiness," and in most cases it is! Making firm decisions is part of being an awesome boss. This is true follow-through.

You need to be a boss to yourself first before you can ever be a boss to anyone else. Having firm, decision-making abilities is truly the difference-maker in having a fulfilling, successful life.

Dealing with Setbacks

Giving up your harmful habits or distancing yourself from toxic people may feel like a loss. We've relied on these coping mechanisms, however unhealthy, for most of our lives. Many of these habits are ingrained in us. Getting over loss (loss of a person, a part of yourself, or a coping mechanism) is a multilevel process.

To begin recognizing and changing your harmful habits, figure out your *Why*. To help to figure out the reason for the habit, it's helpful whenever you catch yourself about to perform a bad habit to simply ask yourself, "Why?" Each time you answer yourself honestly, ask yourself Why again. Do this until you reach the very core of your truth and there are no more "Whys" left to ask.

For instance, often when we think we're busy, we're actually overworking. This harmful habit may seem impossible to quit overnight, since we rely on being busy for our self-worth. When we ask ourselves *Why* we overwork, we may realize that we like the feeling of control when our days are jam-packed and scheduled. But overworking can often lead to illness or strained personal relationships. It's important to remember to continue to ask yourself *Why* you're working so hard. What feeling are you after? What is your core need?

Perhaps you've come to the conclusion that you work so hard because you like to provide for yourself and your family. You're after the feeling of security. However, because you're always working, you don't actually get to spend the quality time with your family that you'd like. Therefore, your relationship with your spouse and children is strained and you never wind up actually achieving your feeling of security. Once you've answered your *Why*, you may realize that despite all your hard work, your needs are not even being met.

If your harmful habit is overworking, you can start by taking an honest look at your schedule. Are you scheduling time for self-love, breaks, and vacations? Can you take a day off and spend it with your spouse? Do you have time to leave work early to plan a special day with your kids? Is there a friend you can reach out to who had similar circumstances and solved them?

The answer is always yes. We *always* have time for ourselves. There is often someone out there who has experienced something similar and can become our council. You filled up that schedule to feel security, and yet it's never delivered the security you've been seeking. Pushing away the pain is, at most, a temporary option. You must gather the *willingness* to realize you need to take time for what's important to you, the *intuition* to embrace that "aha!" moment of recognizing that you are not feeling the security you're after, the *love* to take a different path in the future, and the *discipline* to make time for yourself. If you need a break, take one, but taking too much time off can lead to a depressive episode, or worse, losing your job. Stay inspired. Don't ever stop working on yourself. Don't let setbacks take away your entire life. Keep smiling, keep laughing, and remember: The world is still spinning.

Putting yourself first is extremely important. If you haven't figured this out by the time you start to improve, it can be a great time to begin. Eat healthy, practice some yoga, work out, and get out of the house. You're still here. Life's waiting for you to make the most of it.

Don't shut people out. One of the first things I did after a few days of phone-off, bedridden withdrawals was to reach out to my dear friends and loved ones, many of whom I had no idea had experienced similar situations to mine! This is where I found a lot of my comfort and coping mechanisms.

I have worked harder on myself since I came off my medication than I have ever before in my life. I have also felt the most secure and been the most comfortable. I have acquired the greatest spiritual and personal wealth. This was, for sure, a positive result of recognizing my harmful habits and replacing them, one by one, with WILD habits.

When we lose a harmful habit, there may be a feeling of grief. Grief is messy and confusing and comes and goes in waves like a roller-coaster ride. One of the most powerful things I learned is that grief is a completely natural response to loss, even if that loss is of a harmful habit. Your brain actually has to process *what is not*, which is much harder to process than *what is*. We grieve because we loved, and the loss of love is hard. Grief is a feeling in the process of moving onto a place of healing, but it's not the whole process.

Whether you write about your experience, give back to a cause in someone's name, or somehow share your experience in an empowering way, make the most of what you're going through. What feels like the end of something is often a new beginning. When one door closes, sometimes a whole other house is built, just waiting for you to stop by and make a home.

Intense Commitment

Henry Ford wanted to make a car for the family man. His first "car" (if you can really call it that) had been made while working for the Edison Illuminating Company. It was called the Ford Quadricycle and was literally an ethanol-powered engine with four bicycle wheels mounted on it. Edison saw Ford's vehicle experiments and approved. Standards were pretty low back then. We're talking the late 1890s.

Less than ten years later, Ford had his own company, The Ford Motor Company, and a new mission. Henry Ford declared, "I will build a car for the great multitude. It will be large enough for the family, but small enough for the individual to run and care for. It will be constructed of the best materials, by the best men to be hired, after the simplest designs that modern engineering can devise. But it will be so low in price that no man making a good salary will be unable to own one—and enjoy with his family the blessing of hours of pleasure in God's great open spaces."

This announcement was received with intense skepticism. The general comment was:

"If Ford does this, he'll be out of business in six months."[5]

His haters had a bit of a point. To accomplish his goal, Mr. Ford had to revolutionize the entire automobile industry. Ford Motor Company relied mostly on customer feedback to design the Model T—now considered the most affordable and famous car on the planet. But how was this to be achieved?

His earliest cars were hand-built, one by one, and production was very expensive. To cut costs, Ford started with efficiency. He had a manager time each step that each employee made. He then added up how long each worker was taking to walk from one task to another, and found that many hours were being wasted by men leaving their workstations to find various automobile parts. This simply wouldn't do.

Ford began reducing his employee's tasks by bringing the product parts to them on a moving line so that not a single worker had to leave their station at any point to obtain an automobile part.

Ford's motto was, "Everything can always be done better than it is being done." Hardly a week passed by without some improvement made in the manufacturing process at Ford Motor Company. The company continued to focus on efficiency. Changes happened so quickly, in fact, that they were not even written down. This was a true upset in traditional quality control and management, where every minute change was previously recorded for posterity.

This is how Henry Ford conceptualized the first automobile assembly lines, which allowed production to occur in a more organized, efficient and timely manner. Ford's new concepts meant a large upset in traditional production, but he stuck to his gut. When anyone told him that his "affordable car" was a pipe dream, he did not give up hope. Henry Ford made several models of his car before the Model T. Models A, B, C, N, R, S, and K were all built slightly differently and released at various price points, based on customer feedback. The Model T had practically no features that were not contained in one of the previous models built.

The first Model T left the factory September 28, 1908.

Ford's intense commitment to lowering costs allowed the price of the touring car version of the Model T to be lowered from $850 in 1908 to less than $300 in 1925. On May 26, 1927, Henry Ford proudly watched as the 15 millionth Model T Ford rolled off the assembly line at his factory in Highland Park, Michigan. By that time he had reformed the entire transportation industry and changed millions of people's lives. He is now considered the godfather of the assembly line and mass production, methods that revolutionized the entire Western world by making various commodities affordable. He also helped to birth a new breed of Americans: the middle class.

As he tells us in his autobiography, *My Life and Work,* many years after establishing the Ford Motor Company, Henry Ford had nearly exactly the same number of employees as when he began, despite the demand for his cars being hundreds of times higher! A true testament to his *willingness, intuition, love* and *discipline.* Ford's famous slogan at the time was, "When one of my cars breaks down, I am to blame!" He personally took on this responsibility when he decided to build the universal car; a burden that none of his competition would dare to bear. Ford had tons of critics, including his business partners, good friends, investors, rival inventors, and even his old boss, Thomas Edison. If Ford had allowed the opinions of others to sway him and simply gone about manufacturing traditionally, we might all still be riding in horse and buggies, unable to afford the luxury of a car!

Remember, intense discipline and commitment to your WILD habits can help you follow through with even your wildest dreams and goals.

Confidence in Your Purpose

Your friends and family may be in complete harmony with your purpose, or they may not. You should not allow their stance on your life to discourage you from anything you're passionate about.

When you have an idea, there is a feeling associated with it. When we're inspired, our bodies react to that inspiration and produce high levels of serotonin, dopamine, and oxytocin—our happy chemicals. You get this brilliant idea for a new WILD habit and you ride the wave of it! You write it down, you practice for it, you meditate on it, and you feel grateful for it before it begins!

This creative idea may be a passion project or a hobby you'd love to reignite. It may make no sense to anyone other than you. And that's great! Before the Ford Model T was invented, the eight previous models were tried, sold, tinkered with, and improved. It hardly ever happens overnight or on the first try. Commitment is the key.

Then you finally take the leap and share the idea with someone close to you. Taking this leap means a lot to you. When that person shares his or her opinion with you, it may be positive or negative. Often, it's not the reaction we expect, exactly. This opinion of our idea may be far off base from our own thoughts on it. It is not the opinion, but how you *react* to that opinion that makes the difference. This is one of the most frightening things you can do, because people are bound to have strong opinions. You will have to use your intuition to discern if the opinion is harmful or helpful. Is this person discouraging you because of their own negativity, or are they offering constructive criticism that you can use to help make your idea more viable?

The ultimate experience is one that challenges and changes you. Do you want to live based on other people's opinions of who you should be, or do you want to make a difference in the world?

Your confidence cannot be destroyed unless you truly believe some-one else's opinion of you.

Practicing the WILD Method at Your Breaking Point

Life is hardest when you feel like giving up. This is also when you find your breaking point. These are the times you can do things differently. You can refuse to accept any less than what you deserve. You deserve everything you want, as long as your intentions are pure.

Whenever you hit a roadblock in your personal mission, return to the WILD Method.

Take a moment and acknowledge your willingness. Have you been cutting yourself off from experiences, or have you been shaping your life? What circumstances have brought you here? Are you willing to change them?

Take a moment to listen to your intuition. Let it guide you to hon-esty. Are you truly understanding how life is unfolding for you, or have you begun to allow others to take the wheel? Are you doing what you want to do, or what other people want you to do?

Take a moment to feel true love. Feel true love for yourself first. If you find it hard to forgive or let go, if you find it difficult to deal with someone, ask yourself if you are loving yourself to the best of your ability. When we are in an ultimate state of self-love, judgment and anger disappear. You will find that the more you practice love, the more love you see, feel, and are able to experience. Love is always there. We have to tune into the frequency of it.

Finally, *ask yourself if your persistent willpower (your discipline) is there.* Are you practicing determination or have you given up? Maybe you started some great habits while practicing the WILD Method but found they dropped off after two weeks or so. Maybe you forgot to reorder your supplements. Maybe you forgot to work out on Tuesday, Wednesday, AND Thursday.

Don't give up.

As you will learn in this book, failure is part of the process. We grow more from our failures than our successes—that is, if we learn from them and change our actions the next time we encounter a challenge. As long as we have the patience and willpower to succeed, we have everything we need.

Willpower is a persistent habit. It is an important part of the WILD Method: *discipline in action.*

Go the extra mile—and keep going. Once you start, you'll find it hard to stop. With the knowledge that your plan is sound and your mind is on target, you'll accomplish goals beyond your wildest dreams. You'll find your purpose and follow through on making your dreams your reality. You'll find your self-reliance. You'll feel a sense of ultimate peace—one that cannot be changed by any event, circumstance, or person. Discipline is the direct result of good habits. Once you've mastered discipline, you'll find your core needs are constantly being met. The money materializes. The job presents itself. Exciting opportunities and new friends come knocking. Miracles and synchronicity appear everywhere.

Ask, and you'll start to receive.

How One Mom Decided NOT to Give Up!

Sara had almost given up. Two years after giving birth to her second child, she was facing a body she didn't recognize at all. Early mornings were spent wrangling two high-energy, picky toddlers, with little to no time to begin thinking about her own nutritional needs. She felt she'd tried everything to lose the weight, but with two children to care for starting early in the morning, Sara felt as though she never had the time or energy to exercise. She had tried every diet you can name. Her library was filled with diet and health books, but it seemed she could only stick with her plan for a week or two, and then she would always lose her motivation and fall off the wagon.

Sara finally gave herself the time to recognize her "Why." Sara indulged in harmful, unhealthy eating habits as a method to cope with stress. Her lack of exercise, lack of motivation, and lack of commitment to change had been comfortable for her. Instead of disrupting this harmful habit, for years she'd been masking her pain and stress with more of the same. Focusing on her weight and her body in a negative, defeatist way had drained her mentally, physically and emotionally.

The answer was to address Sara's core needs. Her core need to was to be a healthy person and a good mother. She wanted to be in good shape so she could focus on being the best parent for her children. Sara was sick and tired of hating her body and being frustrated with her appearance. She wanted to focus on being a good role model for her kids. She was done with excuses.

Using the WILD Method, we accessed Sara's *willingness* to change. I asked Sara to picture her life if she didn't change: Where would she be two months, two years, and ten years from now? Sara confessed to me that based on her weight gain in the last two years alone, her *intuition* told her that if she didn't get her weight under control, in a decade she might not be here at all! That scared her, but it also inspired her to take *loving* actions toward herself for the sake of her two children. She made a plan and got *disciplined* about following it.

Sara had read countless self-help and diet books, but she had never given herself the opportunity to actually apply what she had learned. She never had the Willingness to change, the Intuition to listen to her body, the Love to act differently, or the Discipline to stick with a plan. She lacked the WILD Method for a long time. That was all about to change.

Sara began by changing the way she interacted with her children. Instead of getting frustrated with the high energy of her children in the morning, Sara started a new ritual: taking them outside to play. Whether it was a walk to the park, a hike to get coffee, or a play-date with a friend, this got the family's energy out first thing in the morning. With her children down for a nap by noon, she was able to get more done. This left room for exercise, beauty rituals like baths and luxe face masks, and prepping healthy meals—all activities Sara felt she never had time for before. By turning her morning frustration into a WILD habit, the habit of movement, Sara found herself in much better spirits. Because she was constantly moving and had the time to prep healthy meals, her weight naturally and organically came off over the course of a few months. She looks better, feels better, and even got her husband in on their new activity on weekend afternoons! Her family, in turn, has gotten healthier as well.

This is a powerful example of using the WILD Method to your advantage, even when it seems impossible to change. One small shift and a little determination can vastly improve your whole life.

Mastermind Tribe

With this book, you gain a Mastermind Tribe. You can literally reach out to me any time or join our community at The Organic Life. I love hearing from people who read my books. I love learning about your experience and improving myself based on your wonderful words. I've met so many incredible people through practicing, researching, and educating others about the WILD Method. You've all changed my life.

Ideas are like plants: Water them and they'll grow. Once you form a group of people who have similar ideals to you, you can begin to make bigger plans. The power of your mind becomes multiplied as you bounce around ideas, gain inspiration, and brainstorm with one another. You can also connect with other people who've read this book using #WILDHabits on social media. There, you can find a tribe who will support and stimulate you. This is the best way to remind yourself that *no one person knows everything.* The more we educate one another, the stronger we become.

To counteract life being so curated and fake, we have to be wild and free. To balance the times when the world is dark and unnerving, we have to be centered and positive. We have to start sharing our ideas instead of simply repeating or reposting memes of what others have said. We have to tap into our unique creativity.

The fact that you can create means that you should. This is the most unique gift we have. There is no mathematical equation that adds up to humans being the most intelligent, capable, artistic species on earth. It's not a given in any way, but there must be a reason that we are capable of creating so many beautiful things. Look around you: Almost everything, from the chair you may be sitting in to the roof above your head and the book or device you may be holding to the audio you may be listening to, was crafted by someone. From cave paintings to *The Last Supper.* From crude, ancient holes poked into bone and mammoth ivory to the masterful grand piano. From teepees to the incredible, freestanding leaning Tower of Pisa. Creativity is a souvenir for being human. It's a present. Don't ever give this special gift away.

Above All, Practice Love

I had a friend who worked hard for two years to get an investment in his company. Without it, they were bound to go bankrupt.

Finally, after twenty-six months of blood, sweat, and tears, a miracle occurred: An investor put two million dollars in his business bank account overnight. He had every penny he needed to get out of debt, revamp the company, and even rebrand if they wanted to! And with lots of money left over to pay staff and fix margin errors.

Problems solved, right?

The same week that his money went through, my friend received a call that his dad had cancer. The doctor gave his father two weeks to live. He survived for only one of them.

The money, my friend told me, reminded him of all the time he'd spent away from his dad. He'd been too busy making money to spend time with his father while he was around. He had traveled the country, spent countless hours on the phone and on emails, and stalked investors on social media.

My friend felt so guilty about having the money that in six months, it was all gone. Every penny spent—and the company had nothing to show for it. This hadn't solved his problem either, and within months he lost his position in the company altogether.

Without love, all of the joy is taken out of your accomplishments. Be sure you're getting equal love as you are doing hard work. Love needs you as much as you need it. Without love, we may have all of the possessions, money, and power in the world, but we will still be sad, sick, and lonely. Be sure to incorporate plenty of love in your life while you are implementing your new WILD habits.

Your relationships with the people you love are the greatest possessions you own.

The Green Light

Your subconscious mind doesn't know the difference between a day and a year. It doesn't pick up on what's actually real versus what we're allowing ourselves to experience. Time means nothing to your subconscious. It may as well not exist at all. Your subconscious doesn't rely on anything or anyone to tell it what to do, except for you.

Whatever story we tell ourselves is the story we'll live. You could work hard for fifty years and not accomplish what you're able to accomplish in five years, as long as you remain inspired. Your life has a meaning if you voluntarily influence yourself in a positive way. Make sure you're always moving forward and never staying stagnant or moving backward. Propel yourself with the faith that the world has a unique place for you. Through the WILD Method, you can fine-tune and strengthen what that meaning is.

People rarely get this opportunity, but you do! Recognize that by putting in the hard work today, you're making room for a better tomorrow. Give yourself a small goal and watch yourself tackle it, then surpass it. Everything can be yours once you recognize your power.

When you stop your car at a stoplight, you have to wait for the light to turn green for your turn to go. If you drove forward every time someone else's light was green, traffic simply wouldn't work. You have to wait until YOUR light turns green. Making one person's goal a reality right now may delay another person's dream for a moment, but we can all have our time to shine if we are patient and persistent. That's how the green light works to our advantage. It may be frustrating to watch other people succeed and have their moment, but when the light turns green for us, we can totally gun it.

Goal accomplishing can feel easy. Hard work can be fun. Life can be wonderful. We are always connected to the infinite intelligence that allows us to communicate our intention to the universe—and then watch it come to life.

The WILD Method in Action

Condition your mind to work for you while you're sleeping. Play the audio version of this book at night before bedtime. Just before you hit the hay, write a clear statement of what you'd like to accomplish during the next day. Then, read that statement aloud in the morning before you start your day.

It should be something simple and easily doable that propels you toward your goals. Maybe you need to answer an email that may lead to an amazing opportunity. Perhaps you've felt "called" to go for a run but kept putting it off. Now's the time to do it!

Next, set yourself up for success every night by using the WILD Method. Be *willing* to have a more successful day tomorrow. Allow your *intuition* to lead you to your goals. You know you've wanted to run more for ages, and now you're willing to take the *self-loving* action to actually get up a little earlier and do it. To accomplish that run in the morning, it might help to put your running gear out the night before, in addition to setting an alarm. It's both a reminder and an inspiration to suit up and head out. Then when you wake up, instead of throwing on a robe, slip on those running shoes and check yourself out in your athletic apparel first thing in the morning. You'll feel silly *not* going for a run!

Then, form a personal group of more than two people who are on your team and want what's best for you, either in person, at TheOrganicLifeBlog.com, or by using hashtag #WILDHabits. Share this book with them and engage in a friendly discussion about it when they are done. Be sure to encourage one another. If they can't finish or have no interest in self-improvement at this time, maybe they're not meant to be on your team right now. That's okay. Move on and find someone else.

This is your *discipline* in action. Once that goal is accomplished (for instance, once that run is done and you find that buddy to run with you or to send you encouraging morning texts), feel free to come back, check it off, and write a new or improved future accomplishment each night. So if your original goal was to go on a run, your improved future accomplishment could be to go for a run five days a week.

Finally, follow the habit of being more pleasing and joyful than you need to be. Be happier and more pleasant than anyone expects you to be. This is how you get from life exactly what you desire.

⟨❧❧❧❧⟩

Remaining committed to eliminating your harmful habits and replacing them with new WILD habits can be challenging at times. Find a new tribe of people who will support you in practicing the WILD Method for a healthier life. Believing in yourself and ignoring negative comments from others will help keep you on track. As you'll see in Part II, your mindset is your most powerful ally in changing your habits.

PART 2

WILD MIND

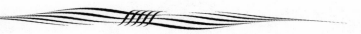

CHAPTER 5

The Miracle of Your Mindset

We all play the victim at one point or another in our lives. Yup. Even you. Sorry. We all do it. A part of us can't help it—it's our ego. We blame our parents for our shortcomings. We blame our spouse for our unhappiness. We blame our siblings for our low self-esteem. Sometimes we even blame ourselves when nothing is actually our fault (usually to elicit some form of sympathy from others).

This is our victim mentality, also called a victim complex. It's a harmful habit, probably one of the worst. The victim desires being a martyr for his or her own sake, seeking persecution and suffering because it satisfies a deeper emotional need—the desire to avoid responsibility. They are victims for the sake of being victims.

A victim mentality is undesirable for two major reasons. First, it keeps people from seeing and acting on the correct choices, which could propel their lives in their intended direction. By focusing on and complaining about what we don't have, by pointing the finger at other people or by blaming someone else for our problems, we're suppressing our own ability to grow, change, and become better. We're giving negativity all the power. Every single moment that we focus on something bad, we are losing the precious moment that we had to focus on something good. Second, by giving in to this mentality, we're attracting more of the same. Think of a victim mentality like building a home: Each thought is a nail in the wood. A victim mentality is rooted in your beliefs and, ultimately, your habits. If you allow words like "I don't," "I can't," "I hate," or "this is awful" out of your mouth, you are hammering those thoughts into your mental home. Likewise, if you replace those negative and victim-based thoughts with thoughts that propel and motivate you, you are setting up a positive mental foundation and your actions will be more loving, positive, and uplifting as well. It's all about changing your mindset to support your WILD habits instead of your harmful ones.

Don't Allow Others' Opinions To Weaken Your Mindset

When I announced some of my goals early in life, I was told by many people that they were unrealistic and couldn't happen. After I announced my lofty dreams, I was informed that I had limitations. When I refused to narrow down a major creative interest, I will never forget what I was told: "Tara, you have to pick *one* thing." When I wanted to move across the country, record music, write a book, or start a company, I was lectured that I didn't have the resources or experience.

I came to realize that I had put hundreds of limitations on myself throughout my life. These limitations weren't facts, but other people's opinions of what I was capable of—opinions that I had internalized, acted on, and built habits from, and that influenced my mindset. Opinions can't be trusted. Opinions, like people, change. Opinions often change based on our *perception* of a situation, not based on the facts.

Did you ever hear something bad about someone from a friend, but then meet the person that friend was complaining about and found that you had absolutely no problem with her? *Hey,* you might think, *Jeana's not so bad after all! What the heck was Marnie talking about?* Your friend was projecting her experience of that person onto you, but you may have an entirely different experience. This is the power of opinion. We are all susceptible to being influenced by the opinions of our friends, families, and significant others, but it's important to remember that we all have a different purpose in life and what may hold one person back may not in any way prevent another from realizing their goals or developing certain friendships.

It is a fact that I had disadvantages growing up, but it was an opinion that my past would limit me. It was a fact that I had many creative interests; it was an opinion that I would have to "pick one thing." It was a fact that I wanted to move across the country; it was an opinion that I wouldn't find the resources to make it work. Once you start to differentiate for yourself the difference between facts and opinions, life will become easier for you, because you can stop listening to and believing other people's negative, limiting beliefs and instead shift your mindset to believe in your own strengths. Sometimes what seem like disadvantages are truly the luckiest and most incredible things that can happen to us, because they provide us with an opportunity for growth or introduce us to new people or situations that will ultimately be beneficial in our lives.

We are the only ones who set the stage for how others perceive us. We can set the bar however high or low we want to, every single moment of our lives. We accept the kind of judgment that exists in our life experience. If we have the right *mindset,* we can easily switch gears from negative to positive thinking and begin to create an automatically positive life.

Once I began to achieve things I had never even dreamed of before, other people's opinions of me changed rapidly. They no longer doubted my ability to accomplish a new goal but instead believed that I would be successful. They expected success. They looked forward to positivity. Be willing to act positively and you'll attract positive people, cultivate positive experiences, and reform your old life into a brand-new one.

Become a Creator

Victims make excuses. Creators make solutions. Victims manufacture problems. Creators produce results. Victims assign blame. Creators take responsibility. Victims focus on faults. Creators imagine perfection. It feels so much better to be a creator than it does to be a victim.

We can build a brand-new mental home by transforming our mindset, ignoring the negative opinions of others, and using the WILD Method to believe in ourselves and our ability to change. We only need to replace our victim mentality with our creator mentality. There are simple solutions to accomplishing this goal. The first lies in changing our language.

For example, if you catch yourself in the habit of thinking unpleasant, negative, or self-deprecating thoughts, you can instantly switch them. This is the basis of neuroplasticity—the ability to rewire your brain and reroute your thinking. I know it sounds simple, maybe even *too* simple to be true. Do you want to know the most amazing secret? Many of the most life-changing and effective truths are incredibly, undeniably simple.

Neuroplasticity habits have already gotten you here. To read and understand this book you've had to learn and repeat many positive habits. You've had to focus on your alphabet, learn your sentence structure, and master your language. In doing so, you've learned to read and understand. Along the way your brain has been your ally, building neurons, structuring memory, and replacing old, irrelevant information with new information. Chances are you no longer say "Da-da" for your father or "Ba-ba" when you want something to drink. Your brain has adapted and improved over the course of your life. Rerouting our negative thinking to positive thinking works in the same way. You need to repeat and practice new, positive thoughts until you have completely replaced your old, outdated language and thought patterns.

Every time you were learning the constructs of language, you were not concurrently learning the intricacies of math. The brain can only focus on one subject at a time. In fact, the brain can only focus on one *thought* at a time. Therefore, every time you focus on something negative, you completely lose that moment to focus on something good. Conversely, every time you choose to focus on positive, uplifting things, you're training yourself to ignore the negative. I promise that if you just try some of these neuroplasticity habits for yourself, you'll see the difference reflected in your own life and day-to-day experience. *Shift your world by shifting your mindset.* Here are some everyday examples:

- VICTIM MENTALITY: "I am terrible at this!"
  CREATOR MENTALITY: "This is difficult but challenges me to learn something new. I will be so proud once I have this down!"

- VICTIM MENTALITY: "I want to do better, but I'm afraid I will fail."
  CREATOR MENTALITY: "The only failure in life is not trying. I can definitely do better and better every day! It will lead me to true fulfillment and success!"

- VICTIM MENTALITY: "I am predisposed to being this way. It is pointless to change because I'll never be perfect."
  CREATOR MENTALITY: "Perfection is not the goal. Balance is the goal. Regardless of any circumstance, I can accomplish any goal. Many people who are more disadvantaged have done it—and so can I!"

Danzi's Mind Reformation from Victim to Creator

Danzi was born in a halfway house and grew up there for the first decade of her life. It was at that halfway house that Danzi's parents' live-in counselor began sneaking into Danzi's room at night and touching her inappropriately. She was threatened, like most victims are, not to tell anyone. These were her very first memories. It took Danzi many years to realize that this had most likely been going on her entire life, and it was not normal in any way.

Finally, on her thirteenth birthday, she decided to speak up about the years of sexual abuse. Once she did, it tore her family apart. Both of her parents blamed themselves. They couldn't believe that the one person they had trusted at the halfway house had betrayed them in such an unimaginable way. Their entire lives were turned upside down, and they had absolutely no support to help them cope. Danzi's mother had a mental breakdown, and both of her parents relapsed. Not long after Danzi came forward about being abused, they both died of drug overdoses within months of each other.

"The guilt I live with every day is paralyzing," she wrote to me. "Before I found your book, I was considering taking my life, too. I didn't know how much longer I could go on with my whole family gone. I have to thank you because your work and your story saved my life."

"But Tara," Danzi continued in her email, "how do I get over this completely? It's been eleven years since they died. I don't have a single happy childhood memory, which is not something many people can relate to. That's why I'm writing to you. For some reason, I feel like you get it. I know you do."

She was right. I did. And I agreed to meet with her in person to see if I could help.

During our meeting, Danzi told me she felt like she was "born depressed, had grown up depressed, and was chemically unstable."

However, she'd been on and off antidepressants for years without any real turnaround. Sometimes it seemed like they helped her get out of bed, she told me, but beyond that she wasn't motivated to even eat three meals on most days.

"Is there a shortcut to happiness?" she asked me. "Or, like, a fast track?"

I laughed and said, "Definitely a fast track, but no shortcuts. You have to put in the work, but honestly, it becomes so rewarding that it truly doesn't feel like work. Happiness is a lifestyle that you can adopt. How long are you thinking?"

"I'd like to be a completely different person by this time next year."

I asked her, "What motivates you? When you get up in the morning, what do you get up and do first?"

"I make coffee and take a walk, put my headphones in, and listen to some music for a few hours, just taking in the neighborhood."

"How does that make you feel?" I prompted.

"A little bit better every day."

"Happiness lies in your purpose. So when you have a purpose, even if it's to get up and make some coffee and go take a walk, you're motivated to get out of bed. Let's expand that. What motivates you in life in general? Why do you feel like you're here?"

When I asked Danzi these questions, she said, "I am the last person left in my family. That's what really keeps me going most days."

Isn't that amazing?

Of course, it's natural that Danzi would miss her family and maybe even carry around a sense of guilt. But for a moment, she can allow gratitude to take over and consider how amazing it is that *she's still alive*. She beat every single odd, and trust me, there were many.

Even though Danzi lost her entire family, she is alive and here on this earth and she can achieve anything she wants. She is not her past or her biography. She is a clean slate at every moment. Each breath is a new chance. She was created for a divine purpose and had lived through every devastating obstacle.

"You *are* a part of your family, but you don't have to live your family's lives," I said to Danzi. "Even if every single solitary family member before you chose a destructive path and a terrible ending, you're still standing here. You're a legacy. You're a legend. You can make a different choice. You can become the example, instead of the tragedy. They get to live on *through you,* but they are *not you.* There is no one else who can carry on what that legacy and legend means *except for you.*"

Those who lack solid family figures in their lives like Danzi may feel their life standards are set low or perhaps were never set at all. They may feel like their parents never taught them anything, such as how to be social, manage money, or eat healthy. Honestly, though it may not seem like it, there is an advantage to Danzi's situation: She can set her own expectations. She can shape her life, her dreams, and her destiny in any way she pleases. The only expectations of who she is or who she should be comes from her alone. She *can* be a completely different person by this time next year—even by this time next week—once she recognizes that nothing is standing in her way except herself.

We all have this capability. Many of us face the daily noise and interference of the opinions of others, so we have a difficult time seeing the power we possess to set our own standards. But at any point you can choose to take advantage of your problems. It's possible that there's a positive way to see the worst situations in your life, whatever they may be. If you've lost someone, it's always going to hurt that they're not here. But in a way, they do live on *through you*. Through every breath and every positive action that you take to get your life in a place where they would be proud of you, you succeed. If you're going to constantly think about your parents, I can tell you that it feels much better to live *inspired by* someone than to live *for* them. There's no validation to having trials and tribulations in life if you don't make something good out of them.

Danzi got busy reforming her mindset and her victim mentality. She completely made over her life and became a creator. She went from seeing herself as a victim to seeing herself as a unique force for positive change. It had taken just a slight shift in mentality for Danzi to begin to shed other people's opinions of who she was and to begin seeing her true self.

Danzi didn't have to change much, other than the one thing that really needed to change: her mindset. She needed to be willing to see things differently, and she finally let go and did. No one had seen the things she had seen. No one had experienced the things she had experienced. No one had suffered exactly the way that she had suffered. And that gave her a one-of-a-kind story, a rare journey, and a lot of life knowledge to begin with. Her tragic background, when used as an education for future experiences, actually gave Danzi an emotional advantage when she decided to view it through a positive light.

Her family and her story still motivates her today, but instead of being a negative story she tells herself, Danzi has used these facts about her life as leverage. She harnessed the power of the creator mentality versus the victim mentality. People had formed many opinions on what Danzi was capable of, but as far as she was concerned, they were all wrong. It was a fact that she had grown up in foster care, but it was an opinion that her upbringing would disable her. It was a fact that Danzi had not learned many coping mechanisms growing up; it was an opinion that she was unable to deal with her life in a positive, constructive way. It was a fact that Danzi had been molested; it was an opinion that her tragedy would destroy her life.

By controlling her triggers, she had controlled her thoughts. As Danzi began to discover that kindness and compassion were some of her core values, she decided to start helping other people. She told me it felt good when she gave back, and I could see it in her face. She had a glow about her, looked a lot healthier, and had a bounce in her step that I had never seen before.

After a few weeks of consistent volunteer work at her local YMCA, she was brighter, cheerier, and seemed much more fulfilled. She complained less and had less time to dwell on her own negative story, which often paled in comparison to the stories of some of the people she was helping every day.

In just a few weeks, Danzi used the WILD Method to overcome her greatest fears and challenges. She had a *willingness* to change in order to cultivate more happiness in her life, and her *intuition* encouraged her to reach out to me for help. Through our conversations and reframing her mindset into a more positive, creator mentality, she learned to *love* herself and to focus more on the activities, such as volunteering at the YMCA, that she loved and that nurtured her passion. And she remained *disciplined* in her pursuit of a happier life and in using her traumatic past as a catalyst for growth. After finally recognizing her true calling, she decided to go back to school, and eventually landed her dream job. Today Danzi is a counselor for foster children. She helps "her kids" (as she affectionately calls them) transition from foster care to new, adoptive homes. Every day she assists in placing children into the kind of homes she always wished for growing up.

"I accomplished my goal—and then some! I am a *completely* different person than who I was that year. And I can appreciate my kids' situations in a unique way," Danzi told me. "I relate to them. I love them, and they love me. Every single time I watch a child find their new home, or I help a parent adopt one of my kids, it makes everything I went through completely worth it. I know exactly why I'm here. I've formed lifelong friendships, and I feel like I'm saving lives by taking these kids out of bad situations, helping to choose the right placement, and making these kinds of transitions easier on everybody. I'm able to do for them what no one was able to do for me."

Danzi's case is extreme, but she has allowed me to share it because it is important for all of us to remember that our past does not define us. Our choices aren't permanent. And we can use our challenging life experiences for our own inner growth, shifting our mindset to see these experiences as opportunities that can lead us closer to our life purpose or path, to becoming creators. Danzi's dearest dream is to open up her own rehab facility, and she is well on her way to doing it. She really feels that this is only the beginning of her journey.

The Law of Manifestation

Willpower isn't just a skill; it's a muscle. Persistence and determination are also powerful muscles. Scientific research has shown that when you become frustrated or disappointed by the outcome of one thing, you are much more likely to quit faster on another task. Your successes build a successful feeling in the same way that exercise builds muscle mass. Conversely, your failures are also more likely to cause future failures. When you fail at something, even one time, you are more likely to carry that feeling of failure with you through the rest of your day, your week—sometimes your whole life. In this way you are building up your failure muscle, instead of concentrating on building up your success muscle.

That is why it sometimes seems so impossible to overcome the feeling of failure, and why many people think that they've been "born unlucky." One bad situation has led to another, which has led to feelings of defeat. We carry these defeatist feelings into the next situation, and the cycle tends to repeat itself. We're all victims of this at one point or another. You must come to recognize that it's a concept that's been following you, perhaps for most of your life. If you don't choose to change your negative state, this is no different than wishing for something bad to happen.

You manifest your outcome through your feelings, not the other way around. Form follows function. What you dwell on, you become. You manifest your outcome. Your circumstance does not define you. If you have already manifested disease, illness, or a chronic problem into your life, your first step is to stop drawing your attention to the problem in a negative way. Disease cannot live in a healthy body; the very word itself (dis-ease) highlights that. Negativity cannot survive in a positive mind. This means that you need to surrender to yourself and switch your attention. What you continue to focus on, you will create more of, which means that if you focus on the problems in your life, you will only receive more of them. It also means that if you focus on healing, positive thinking, and taking control of your body, you will receive more healing and your life will reflect your positive mindset. You will gain more peace, serenity, and control over your body and your life. You'll willingly come to possess what you seek and find that you can entirely tame your subconscious mind. This is known as the Law of Attraction or The Law of Manifestation, and it's a scientific miracle when we know how to tap into it to use it to our advantage.

Unfortunately, most people aren't aware that they possess the amazing ability to do so and therefore continue to attract more negativity into their lives by thinking about what they *don't* want instead of what they *do* want. I will teach you how to use this law to your benefit so that you can successfully release your harmful habits and negative mindset and create WILD habits that support the positive changes in your life.

Harnessing Your Thoughts

Think of your mind as a river. Each droplet in the river is another thought you have. From far away the river seems to be solid, but look closer and you'll see that in reality it's an ever-changing, growing flow. The river is constantly purifying itself, endlessly flowing and filtering what it does not need or cannot support. It has slow seasons and busy seasons where there's spawning, fishing, or feeding. Sometimes the river is frozen completely. Come spring, it always thaws.

Just as the river does this, you can also do this with your mind. Your consciousness is constantly evolving. You do not have the same thought process now as you had when you were an infant or when you were seven years old. It's probably not even the exact same one as you had last year or maybe even last week! If you want to change anything about yourself, you need to start with your thoughts. Begin by changing the process that is likely subconscious and that leads to a habit of negative thinking.

Oh, you thought all that negative, repetitive thinking was just you? Nope. You've got company. It seems that humans have somewhere between 12,000 to 60,000 thoughts per day,[6] but according to some research, as many as 98 percent of them are *exactly the same* thoughts as we had the day before. Perhaps most significantly, as many as 70 percent of our daily thoughts are negative![7]

Much like how you may wear a hole in your shoes from repetitive walking, you wear holes and paths in your mind with repetitive thoughts, regardless of whether those thoughts are positive or negative. We may feel powerless to our thoughts, and it may even feel like they have complete control over us. But how long have we been thinking like this—helplessly? And how do we stop this behavior in ourselves? We can start by harnessing our thoughts and choosing to consciously focus on the positive ones and release the negative ones.

When scientists first used a PET scan to track thoughts, they noticed that each thought displayed on the screen was a unique universe of its own. When tracked, the thoughts linked to strong smells, memories, or pain sensations reached not just a single site in the brain, but *several* sites in the brain.

We have endless ways to transform our neural pathways and rewire our minds so that we alone create our universe. Wouldn't you like to be able to control your pain, your anger, your habits, or the larger direction of your life? It's entirely possible!

Thoughts are merely mental synapses that have been wired and rewired over time. Your thoughts alone determine your level of failure and success, and your thoughts are easily molded. That is why it is so easy to suspend our disbelief when we watch a movie or TV show. When we allow it to, our brain has the ability to "suck us in," even to things we know very consciously are not real. And yet we truly *feel* for our favorite characters. We laugh at their jokes. We cry at their losses. We feel triumphant at their successes.

Your mind can mold its thoughts at any moment just like clay can be molded into a vase. Clay is pliable, but once it's been fired, it's set. Your mind works this same way: Thoughts are what mold your mind every moment, and these thoughts become your mentality. This mentality then ultimately becomes your personality and your attitude, which is when it "sets." If we go too long with this mentality without ever remolding it or opening ourselves up to new ideas about who we are, our mentality gets "set" this way. That is why it gets harder to change our beliefs as we get older.

Dean Ornish, MD, is the founder and president of the Preventive Medicine Research Institute, as well as a clinical professor of medicine at the University of California, San Francisco. Dr. Ornish has conducted impressive scientific studies that show a reversal of serious heart disease using a combination of meditation, positive thinking exercises, group therapy, walking, and a plant-based diet.

Research has shown that coronary arteries, which feed the heart with blood, can get clogged up with cholesterol and other deposits, much like rust builds up in a pipe. Until recently, it was believed that the best you could do was slow down the process or have risky bypass surgery. However, Dr. Ornish's research revealed that through his program 82 percent of his patients' arteries had become less blocked. In an interview with Bill Moyer in Moyer's book *Healing and the Mind*, Dr. Ornish says:

> As it turned out, we showed that there often was reversal. We found a direct correlation between the amount of overall adherence to the life-style program (of positive thinking, meditation and relaxation techniques) and what happened in the arteries.
>
> Now, unlike most things we do as doctors, the worst that can happen if someone practices stress management, for example, is that they can manage stress better. This is not like putting someone on medications that can have serious side effects, both known and unknown. . . .
>
> . . . Any time a person is in pain, there is an opportunity for a transformation. . . . When people learn to experience inner peace—when we work on that level—then they are more likely to make and maintain life-style choices that are life-enhancing rather than self-destructive. . . . If we can show—as we have in three separate studies—that through life-style

changes alone, not only do people feel better, but they *are* better, then to me, life-style change is a valid alternative to cholesterol-lowering drugs and surgery. And people need to know that they have alternatives.[8]

Control Your Thoughts

It's an old superstition to believe we can't rewire our thoughts or change our destiny. Your past doesn't belong to you, and you don't belong to it. Think of your past like a jail sentence: It cannot imprison you if you don't live in it. True emotional freedom lies in giving up our sad past stories for the sake of making good memories in the present. This helps us both now and in the future.

Until Roger Bannister broke the four-minute mile, everyone thought it was impossible. But once one person did it, it became fairly routine. Your happiness and your destiny is dependent on you. You deserve what you allow yourself to accept. Accept nothing but the best. Control your thoughts and you control your entire life.

Give yourself a breath and start with fresh energy. Don't continue your task until you've changed your physical and mental state. Change your body language. Stand up straight. Breathe deeply and calmly until you feel differently. This type of breathing activates the parasympathetic nervous system, which helps produce a sense of relaxation and contentment. This allows us to be calm and clear when deciding which inspired action to take next.

Smile until you feel better. Pay attention to where you place your focus. According to Vedantic tradition, "Intent is a force of nature." When intention is repeated, we create habit. The more we repeat our intention, the most likely this is to manifest in our physical world. To manifest at the greatest level, we have to quiet our minds and focus on our true beings.

Most people think first and foremost about themselves. They drown in their own misery, get caught up in a victim mentality about their problems, internalize the limitations that others place on them, and throw mini pity parties for every uncomfortable feeling they have. People who live for themselves create a web of negativity that entangles them. It's inescapable. It's science. And science doesn't play favorites. The Law of Manifestation is true physics and it applies to all of us. The law applies whether you are taking positive or negative action. Choose to be a creator instead of a victim and begin to notice the positive people and experiences you attract into your life. Build your willpower muscle, harness your thoughts, and place your focus on successfully incorporating new WILD habits into your life. Choose to place your focus on the positive and watch what manifests in your life.

CHAPTER 6

The Power of Energy

Energy is undeniably real. We know that it has the power to heat, generate, electrocute, and give life, and that it can never be destroyed. Energy runs every machine, from cars to planes, in addition to our atoms and light. It doesn't just propel, react, and regenerate—energy listens. It even listens to you—to your thoughts and emotions. In the previous chapter you learned about the Law of Attraction and how your thoughts can manifest your desires. Now you'll discover how this all ties into energy and what it means to *raise your vibration.*

When energy is absent, inspiration is insurmountable. Without energy, we have no motivation. If we have the energy to go on that run, it's easy. If we don't, it can seem impossible. Without energy, we're likely to succumb to sedentary bad habits that affect our mood, weight, anxiety, and so much more. Our energy levels ultimately determine our fate.

Strong emotions can override other signals in the body. This is how energy listens. All of our thoughts and actions, both conscious and subconscious, have an effect on our energy, and our energy has a huge impact on how we feel every day.

Many of our choices are subconscious, and perhaps rightly so. Bombarding the body with more choices is never the answer to personal growth. Instead, harnessing the choices that we're already making is where all of our answers to freedom and happiness can be found. If we could start to recall what we wanted to recall and feel how we wanted to feel instead of being a slave to our bodies and minds, we could use these exercises every day in order to constantly improve and raise our energy vibration. Learn how to tap into the energy around you and use it to your advantage to create the life of your dreams.

Miracles happen every day. They don't only occur in shrines and they're not just emblazoned numbers on gigantic checks given out on talk shows. Miracles can happen in our health, can show up in our relationships, and are hidden in our opportunities. We must simply harness and control our energy. Then we can sit back and watch miracles unfold.

The Science of Energy

We have a consciousness that exists above and beyond what can be readily observed. For instance, pay attention to your posture in this moment. Are you sitting up straight or are you slouched? Are your legs crossed? Have you been rocking your knee? Is your finger on the next page to turn it? Perhaps all of the above. All of these movements are subconscious, but they affect our energy at every moment. If we don't pay attention to our posture, this can affect our health, giving us arthritis, spinal problems, or chronic pain. If we don't pay attention to our breath, this could lead to unhealthy coping mechanisms like panic, which lowers our ability to handle our problems calmly and correctly. If we don't get ahold of habits like rocking our knee or pacing, they could haunt us long term, affecting us socially, which in turn affects how we deal with and handle the world around us.

Maybe we don't constantly think about if we're smiling when others are talking to us, but if we always speak to someone with a smile, this is how people will always remember us. We don't continually consider where we bear our weight, and yet becoming aware of it can help our health, our breathing, our chi, our spine, and ultimately shape our entire lives. This is how the energy we have helps us become the person we truly are.

Intelligence is present everywhere in our bodies. Your body is always listening. It listens to your words, your actions, and your thoughts. It may seem like the mind and the body are not connected, but let me show you a perfect example of how they're linked.

Imagine for a moment that you have a lemon in your hand. Bring the lemon from your hand up to your nose. Deeply inhale the scent of the lemon. Now cut the lemon. Imagine the feeling of slicing through fruit on a cutting board with a knife. Now, begin to enjoy a slice. Imagine the lemon in your mouth. What does it feel like? What does it taste like?

Chances are, you had a reaction. Either salivation or maybe your mouth puckered, sensing the taste of lemon. Now, ask yourself: *Where is the lemon?* The lemon isn't in your mouth. It's not even in your pocket. If a doctor did an operation, they couldn't find the lemon inside your brain. In truth, the lemon doesn't really exist. But, in fact, you could easily recall a lemon without actually seeing or feeling one. Your body reacted to a lemon just by imagining it.

Use Energy To Manifest Your Goals and WILD Habits

There are powerful ways that you can use your energy to your advantage. Here is one exercise in which I use energy to manifest my goals:

1. Recall a time where you felt accomplished.

2. Now picture a future goal. Maybe you want to be on the cover of *Vogue,* write a best-selling memoir, or be comfortably

living in your dream home. Imagine yourself accomplishing that goal. Picture the very moment it happens.

3. Picture the day your magazine or book hits the shelves. Immerse yourself in the moment you turn your keys and step inside your front door. Get comfortable as you lay in your dream bed. If you have trouble feeling accomplished, carry the feeling of your last accomplishment (the one we pictured at the beginning of this exercise) into this new thought.

4. Allow yourself to feel how you will *really* feel after you accomplish your new goal. Let yourself experience that feeling for five or ten minutes instead of a fleeting few seconds. Bask in that feeling. Go new places in your imagination. Let that feeling overwhelm you. Picture the smile on your face and the feeling of triumph.

5. Carry this new "memory" (remember, our brains don't know the difference between what's real and what's imagined) into your work as you start to accomplish this dream or goal. You'll be surprised how much of what you picture manifests in exactly the way that you have envisioned!

In this way, you're using energy—the power of your imagination—to help you recognize and then proactively fulfill your dreams. Practiced vividly and with conviction, this exercise works to align ourselves with our intention. By imagining our goals as being already accomplished, we begin the process of sending messages out to the universe that *this is what we want*. And just as our energies and our bodies listen, the energy of the cosmos listens, too. Once you carry the belief of your future goal with you, through the power of your own energy other people begin to listen as well. Then those people will happily conspire with you to make your dreams a reality. Once you project those intentions, you secure a place in the world for them to manifest. This is how goal accomplishing works. Once you simply have the *intention*, you're halfway there. Use the WILD Method to develop the awareness needed to reach your goals head on:

- Be *willing* to recognize how your conscious and subconscious choices have shaped you. Are you focusing so much on negative thoughts or beliefs that there is no room for positive ones to manifest?

- Use your *intuition* to address why you've made these choices again and again. What needs were you trying to fulfill? How can you fulfill them in a positive way?

- Approach yourself with the true *love* it takes to forgive yourself and change for the better in the future.

- Keep up the persistent *discipline* in your better decision-making process. This attitude is what's needed to prosper on a long-term basis.

The more often we do this, the closer we are to true emotional success. We live in a world that has a bias toward negativity. To combat this, we need to repeat and reinforce positive actions for ourselves the same way we have repeated negative ones—and to an even greater extent.

We can mess up a few times. No one is expected to be perfect the first time they try to tackle a harmful habit. It's also been proven that the more we fail, the more we learn. Studies suggest that self-experimentation—that is, seeing what works for you—is the best route to long-term success. Instead of failures, think of your mistakes as experiments. If you're going to do an experiment, make sure you are willing to learn from it so you don't have to repeat it.

Once we become aware of our tendencies, we have the power to shift them and make them positive, which immediately has a positive life impact. Refer to the WILD Method mentioned before throughout the day and return to the method any time you feel lost in your path to happiness.

Raise Your Vibration—and Change Your Life

Have you ever searched frantically for something only to have it show up in the last place you looked? Or lost something that you never found until you gave up looking for it? Maybe you tried to force something in your life, but it never seemed to work out until you relinquished control? This is part of the Law of Attraction, and we can use it to manifest the exact life we desire.

Most manifestation occurs when you make up your mind. Once you make a thorough decision about what you truly want out of life, the stage has automatically been set. The majority of the work is done for you—IF you keep your eye on the prize. Commit to your wants and goals. Keep them in the back of your mind, and don't get frustrated if they don't appear immediately. Remember the Green Light: The universe is a vast place; making one person's dream come true may delay another person's dream for a few years. Know that you will have your time if you're persistent and clear on your goals.

Your body knows your intention. You are what you allow yourself to accept. When we get frustrated, our bodies respond to that frustration. It may seem harmless to let stress take over, but accumulation of negative consciousness is where illness and sadness manifest.

There is a magical form of your conscious expression, which says that anything that can be yours will be yours. The universe is always paying attention to your conscious expression.

For the next three weeks I want you to listen *only* to yourself. Raise your vibration by shifting your focus. Do things that bring you joy. Get out your paint set, go for a walk every day, and call your loved ones. Reach out to others. Get proactive about your goals, and indulge in your WILD habits. Be mindful about how you're spending your money and time. Fulfill needs that are not about ego gratification. Plan a trip somewhere you've never been before (even if it's just a picnic at a new park). Eat mindfully and with color on your plate. Act toward yourself like you would act toward your greatest mentor or the person you admire the most. You're not necessarily listening to yourself talk, you're listening to your body—exclusively. Though this might seem selfish at first, it's the most *selfless* thing you can do.

List three ways you're committed to raising your vibration and listening to yourself for the next thirty days. When you do this, mentally explore how these actions will empower you to help others:

How I will raise my vibration:

1. _____

2. _____

3. _____

How that will help me:

1. _____

2. _____

3. _____

How that will help others:

1. _____

2. _____

3. _____

The more you listen to yourself, the more you can listen to, understand, and help others. You'll be able to tune in to your most basic instincts, such as what your body truly needs instead of what you might crave in the moment. We create our reality. Form follows function—not the other way around. You tell your body what to do, and your body will instinctually follow suit, even if that positive action has been drowned out, beat up, or brought down for years.

It only takes twenty-one days to change your entire life, because that's how long it takes to change most of your habits. In less than a month you can move from craving sweets and coffee to not just consuming but enjoying exercise, kale smoothies, chard salad, fermented veggies, healing teas, and more! You can apply this life philosophy to your dinner plate, your job, and your relationships.

In Western culture, many of us have been raised to manifest, but we haven't been taught *how* to do it. Often we're told we are capable of anything, but we're not instructed how to define or reach that "anything." We try to force things to happen instead of guiding them to happen. When you force things to happen, they'll never truly work out.

Nature is not forced, and yet plants respond very well to guidance. I have rescued and adopted plants that previous owners were convinced were dead. And yet simply by potting the plant with the right drainage or soil, talking to the plant, encouraging her, singing to her, and giving her the correct water, sunlight, and nutrients, the plant will almost always miraculously resurrect. Often a plant flourishes in the hands of someone who takes the time to understand her. My friends cannot believe six months later that the healthy, exquisite, flowering tower of orchids in my yard were once the shriveled, dehydrated "dead plant" they had thrown in their trash two seasons ago.

I have witnessed plants die mostly from neglect, especially with timid plant owners convinced that they "don't have a green thumb."

The negative energy from their premature feelings of defeat end up affecting their ability to care for the plant. Plants respond very well to positive energy. Give a plant love, light, and encouragement, move it next to healthy plants, let it know it's safe, and you can clearly see the difference in the way it grows. This has been proven in multiple scientific studies, but perhaps was demonstrated most powerfully in the case of illustrious scientist Luther Burbank, who developed more than eight hundred strains and varieties of plants in his fifty-five-year career.

While developing a breed of spineless cactus, Burbank thought to use an uncommon tactic that many scientists thought of as ludicrous: love. He kindly asked the plants to cooperate with him. The scientist reported that he often talked to his plants, encouraging them, speaking soothingly, and explaining to them how they don't need their spikes to protect themselves. They—that is, the cacti he bred—were said to have helped Burbank in ultimately achieving his goal. "The secret of improved plant breeding, apart from scientific knowledge, is love," he once told a visitor, reiterating his conviction.[9]

If I can resurrect countless dead plants by giving them the right amount of love, sunshine, and nutrients, and Burbank can aid the breeding of a spineless cactus partially by speaking kindly to it, imagine the implication on what kindness and good energy can do for us as humans! A little bit of love, guidance, and encouragement can go a long way. Keeping our energy positive and trusting in the work we're putting in today can have an incredible long-term impact on our future. This involves self-loving actions like meditation, getting outdoors, and practicing mind-strengthening techniques and new, WILD habits. Don't forget to encourage yourself each and every day, despite any odds you may face. One moment lost to a negative thought is bad enough—but a year or a lifetime lost to negative thinking is devastating. We do ourselves a great disservice by not taking our energy seriously. It's up to us to consistently take into account and acknowledge how our energy may be affecting our lives as a whole, so that only positivity and encouragement remain, helping to propel us toward our goals.

When you guide things to happen, they happen naturally and you find true gratification in their success. All you have to do is water the good seeds in your life, step back, and watch them grow.

For the next three weeks, guide your life. Listen to your gut reactions instead of being influenced by outside circumstances or people. Use your intuition. Get disciplined. Pay attention to what you truly want. Stop living life on autopilot, and start taking the wheel.

SIMPLE WAYS TO RAISE YOUR VIBRATION

1. Be conscious of the foods you're consuming. Make sure your plate is colorful: greens, blues, browns, reds, and oranges, too. Enjoy organic, GMO-free food whenever possible. The more organic the food, the higher its vibration (we'll touch more on this subject in chapter eight).

2. Find something beautiful to appreciate. Whether it's a flower, the sunset, or the sound of your own breath, gratitude is a powerful way to raise our vibration because it brings us back to the present moment.

3. Practice random acts of kindness. Smile more than you need to smile. Be kind to everyone you meet. Try throwing preconceptions about people away before interacting with them.

4. Take a Himalayan salt bath. Himalayan salt contains eighty-four minerals in total, making it super high-vibe and great for relaxation and detoxification. Toxins are released from your body while your skin absorbs the healthy minerals into your body.

Express Gratitude

Our experience is merely a representation of what we've attracted and unlocked unconsciously. There is a super-secret way of making sure that the universe not only gets the message but also allows the vibrations you're sending out to work to their greatest potential. The answer lies in being grateful for your new life before it happens. Those who see the largest impact of gratitude in their life are those who understand that the universe is here to work *for* and *with* them. If you think it, you can create it.

Once you're consciously creating your experiences, you're actively taking charge of your reality and your happiness. Anything can happen for you if you use these tools to your advantage instead of allowing other people's manifestations to rule your destiny.

When you are grateful for good things before they happen, you are essentially tricking your body into believing that good things have *already* happened. We trick our bodies like this in some small form every day. Whether we cringe at a gory part in a movie, get excited about a gift before we receive it, or salivate at the thought of food, our bodies are capable of mentally experiencing something *before* we physically experience it.

Apply the WILD Method to find your gratitude and propel your life:

Have the *Willingness* to accept and find grace. Ask yourself what you WANT to be grateful for (even if it hasn't happened yet!). What's the one thing you'd get up every morning and thank your lucky stars for if you had?

Use your *Intuition* to map out your intention. Intention can be so powerful. When we guide our intention in the direction of our dreams, we propel our lives forward at light speed. Make sure that your intention is based on your true purpose and not on what you believe others expect of you. Ask yourself:

- Will my goal truly bring me happiness?
- Am I looking to fill holes missing somewhere else in my life?
- What is the true intention of my goal? Why do I want it?
- What will I do every day to get it?

Adjust your *Intuition* to match your true intentions. Strive to become wise and forthright in *all* your actions—not just forthright in *some* of them. You can apply your newly learned strategies to every area of your life. Be kind in your speech and recognize that other people's energy directly affects your own.

Keep guard of your mind and your emotions. They are the most precious gifts you have. When you react to low energy, you've matched it. You are spreading a cycle of hating someone for hating you, which is not a solution. This creates dis-ease in our minds and our bodies and should always be avoided. If you have the power to recognize low energy, you have the power to rise above it.

When other people are making life difficult or stressful, use your *Love* to show compassion for yourself and them—and keep moving on. Sometimes when we get clear on our goals, toxic people show up to throw us off course. They may even convince our allies to do the same. This is a distraction from our true purpose, which is exactly their intention. Use love and gratitude to battle this. Forget other people's opinions. For example, if you're trying to find a new job, instead of focusing on negativity about the job market, express gratitude for this new position before you even have it.

Discipline is willpower. We have to practice willpower for it to have a lasting effect on our life. When difficult things arise, do you find yourself making the right choice or the comfortable choice? Do you indulge in hate or choose love? Do you seek escape or work through the hard emotions head on? Respect your decision making. Tune into what *feels* right. When you make a decision about what that is, follow through.

Dr. Roy Baumeister is a social psychologist who explores how we think about the self, and why we feel and act the way we do. He's the leading expert in willpower. One of Baumeister's ego depletion studies asked hungry students to resist a plate of freshly baked chocolate chip cookies before trying to solve a puzzle requiring them to focus and draw on their self-control. This group was compared to students who were also asked to solve the puzzle (which was unsolvable, by the way) but who *did not* have to resist the cookies first. As you may have guessed, the students who were asked to resist grew frustrated quicker, had a hard time resisting, and did poorly.

It's harder to focus on a challenging task and exert self-control after you've already used up most of your willpower—especially when it comes to ignoring a plate of warm chocolate chip cookies! The study noted that "choice, active response, self-regulation, and other volition may all draw on a common inner resource."[10] Since that study was conducted in 1998, other studies have found similar results. That "inner resource" the study notes is the basis of our willpower, which touches on nearly all aspects of healthy, abundant living: eating right, exercising, avoiding drugs and alcohol, studying more, working harder, spending less, and saving money. Our discipline *is* our willpower. Like our muscles, the more we practice self-discipline, the stronger our willpower becomes.

The Happiness Habit

Happiness is not earned in any traditional way. If you wait until you "deserve" to feel happy or you feel that you "need a reason" to start thinking pleasant thoughts, your life is likely to continue in its current direction. By waiting to feel happy, we're giving in to guilt—guilt about our worthiness, guilt about our pleasures, and guilt about our selfishness. Most people live this way: waiting to be happy. They don't live life now in the present, but for some happy event they've planned for in the future. They think, "If I get promoted, I'll be happy," "If only I lose some weight, I'll be happy," or "When I fall in love, I'll be happy." Worse, many people spend their here and now pining over some past sad event.

Life inevitably creates a certain set of problems, and if we don't look at those problems as opportunities to grow, we'll only get stuck. The longer we are stuck in a pattern of waiting for happiness, the longer it can take to get unstuck from this expectation. If you are happy at all, you must be happy, period. Not happy "because of" something. This is the happiness habit. Happiness is earned by performing this habit again and again, until it becomes a way of life for you.

Now, you might say, "How can I just conjure up happiness without a reason? If I could do that, wouldn't I have been doing that all along?" Perhaps, but many people *don't even realize* that they carry the tools with them to create happiness.

The Tools to Create Happiness

Some of the most powerful tools to create happiness are right at our fingertips, we're just never taught them. It's like this: Turn the radio to 97.5 and you might hear Christian rock. Turn it to 97.9 and you might hear hip-hop. If you never turn the radio dial, you may think the radio *only* plays Christian rock. Other radio waves are always in the air, but we need to be tuned in to them to hear the correct frequency. In this case, the frequency is your peace of mind, the basis for happiness. If we experience dis-ease, depression, or anxiety, and we never tune in to other ways of thinking and living, we'll always be stuck on the same station, having the same experiences, creating the same situations for ourselves on a seemingly endless loop.

Happiness has less to do with your circumstances than previously thought. In 2013 psychologists from the University of California found that genetics and life circumstances only account for about 50 percent of a person's happiness. The rest is up to you.[11]

Happiness, as we're talking about it here, is an appreciation of one's life as a whole. To appreciate our lives fully, we must be grateful for what we have. Every morning, write down five to ten things you're grateful for. This is your daily gratitude list, a WILD habit that propels your happiness.

My Gratitude List

1. _____

2. _____

3. _____

4. _____

5. _____

Take at least a minute to think deeply about each one. If you wrote "My family," for instance, think about the time you spend with your family and what you love about them. This is your daily gratitude practice. As we touched on earlier, the more you think about the things you're grateful for, the more abundantly you'll receive them. What you focus on grows.

Be sure to start moving more than normal. Getting your body moving for as little as ten minutes releases GABA, a soothing neurotransmitter that also limits impulsivity. Exchange an hour of TV a day for an hour of cardiovascular exercise, which has been proven to decrease stress and increase happiness by increasing serotonin and endorphins. A University of Bristol study revealed that people who exercised on workdays reported improvements in mood, time management, and work performance. Researchers noted, "The effect of happiness on longevity in healthy populations is remarkably strong. The size of the effect is comparable to that of smoking or not."[12]

Tuning back into ourselves is another important tool. Chances are, whatever is depressing you or causing you anxiety has been solved before and lies in the pages of a book, and like this one, millions of books on self-improvement and success have been written. Keep reading. Keep searching to see what others have done during moments of crisis. If you really want to break out of the mundane, expect the impossible. Expect the world to heal and get better. Expect people to soften. Expect the environment around you to be more positive. Only by repeatedly thinking good thoughts do we manifest them into our lives and change the world.

Live your happiness. Make sure happiness is reflected in your posture and your face. What do happy people look like? They smile. They hold their head high, have good posture, and speak confidently. They attract the company of others. They exude a light about them. They make other people feel good. Try to focus on your inner light shining through your eyes, especially when you engage with other people. People will notice the fire and glow in your eyes and always respond more positively to you.

When Warren Buffet and Bill Gates first met, they were each asked to write a word that they felt best described why they'd been so successful over the years. Two of the richest men in the world, without saying a word to one another, wrote down the exact same thing: Focus.

What you focus on grows. If you focus on happiness, living a good life, and being a positive person, you'll attract more opportunities for happiness to show up. You'll attract people who are happy, because happy people keep happy company. Focus on the best version of yourself, on moving forward from tragedy and dis-ease, on being a healthy human, and on living a fulfilling life. Focus on your goals, and one by one, watch your goals manifest into your reality.

Use the WILD Method as a tool to build your happiness habit:

Ask what you're *Willing* to change. Have you been stuck in negative habits or thinking patterns that have hurt you? What are you willing to let go of and how will that serve you in your quest for happiness?

Use your *Intuition* to bring happiness into your life. When were you happiest? What brings you the most joy? Whose company can you keep so that you are always smiling, laughing, and growing? What project, activity, or cause can you immerse yourself in that will make you happiest?

Love yourself without judgment as you are now, then picture yourself at your best. Perhaps it matches up to you today, perhaps you have some room to grow. Hold the image of yourself at your best. See yourself smiling or laughing. Who is around you? Surround yourself now with the light that emanates from you when you are at your healthiest and happiest.

Practice the *Discipline* to not only picture yourself as a happier person but also follow through with these positive, confident actions in your everyday life and actually *become* a happier person.

Don't Give Away Your Power to Be Happy

To a large extent, we're content with reacting unconsciously to petty annoyances. We're used to grumpiness, disappointment, and dissatisfaction. We become accustomed to gut reactions. For instance we honk our horn in traffic, turn on the TV when we're bored, check our phone without a reason, get disappointed in other people, or interrupt someone while they're talking. We've practiced these reactions for many, many years. They're comfortable for us. But they don't build happiness.

The world can be scary, but we have to remember our true place in it. The White House is probably not in your living room. The drama of other people is not your own drama. If we let bad news or the constant anxiety of the media get to us, we give away the power we possess to improve our own lives. These circumstances can only affect us as much as we allow them to. We can turn off the TV anytime (in fact, we can throw our TV in the garbage, where some may argue it belongs). We can choose not to pick up a newspaper, turn the radio to a different station, or donate to causes without letting them take over our life. We can help in a productive way without letting bad news depress us. We give away our power to other people, media, circumstances, events, and our past . . . all the time. Sometimes it may seem easier to give away our power, but it's not helpful in the mission of improving our life. Allowing someone else or outside events to dictate our lives is like being a sheep whose only thought is following her shepherd.

You are not a sheep. But if you follow along like one, eventually you will feel directionless, obedient, and reactive. I call this a slave mentality. When you're in a slave mentality, you're promptly obeying some outside event, circumstance, or person instead of listening to your true self. Often your goals become lost or meaningless, and you wind up angry, sick, upset, and unhappy.

Assess your happiness in this simple, effective way:

- How happy am I now?

- How happy do I want to be?

- What positive actions can I take to get there?

Your positive actions will include your gratitude practice, your daily movement, exercises, time for yourself, meditation (which we'll expand on in the next chapter), your kindness to others, and finding ways to give back. Simply keep an eye out for how you can make each moment into an opportunity for happiness and excitement. When we repeatedly do this, we build our happiness muscle.

The Positive Actions I'll Take to Achieve Happiness

1. _____

2. _____

3. _____

4. _____

How to Build Your Happiness Muscle

Each area of your life will be easier if you get one thing down first: your happiness habit. Every night, keep a mental and physical diary of your habits throughout the day. Write down in a new journal entry the improvements you made when faced with hard choices, negative thoughts, or temptations.

My common daily habits:

1. _____

2. _____

3. _____

4. _____

My daily improvements:

1. _____

2. _____

3. _____

4. _____

Keep a journal—NOT notes in your phone. Not your voice recording device you'll never listen to again. Don't text it to yourself. WRITE it down.

Write any chance you get. It's a completely different muscle, and it is connected to a separate part of the brain than texting or typing. During texting or typing, you are accessing your "tech muscles" (you've memorized QWERTY, how to open an app, how to type, capitalize, and save it).

When you handwrite, you are accessing your creative muscles. Your hands move and your brain *has to remember how to write*. It helps memory recall, comprehension, and conceptual development. Writing is linked to improved memory and creative skills. It helps your critical thinking. By holding the writing instrument, feeling the surface, holding the paper down, and directing the precise movement of your fingers, you improve your fine motor skills by tapping into your neurosensory experience. The act of writing can become your new WILD habit. For instance, writing this book has been a very therapeutic experience for me, as it is for many authors. It helps us engage with ourselves and fuels our connection to the world. Let writing become one of your WILD habits and watch how miraculously it affects your life and your happiness.

When you write, begin to access how you deal with stress and what goals you're working toward. Never identify yourself with mistakes or bad behavior. If you've done wrong, admit you've done wrong and resolve to do better, but don't focus on it. This is the way to overcome your sadness and anxieties head on.

Ask yourself the following questions every day:

1. Did my habits lean toward happiness and positivity?

2. Have I been making the choices I felt were right at the time, or have I been denying my goodwill instincts?

3. Can I try harder to be better?

These three questions, when asked and answered earnestly every night, will guide you in the direction of an incredibly improved life. After handwriting your gratitude and habits list, ask yourself these three questions and then write down the moments you're most grateful for throughout the day. Perhaps someone was kind to you when you least expected it. Maybe your cat cuddled with you while you were sick. Maybe your mom told you how proud she was of you. All of these precious moments can overwhelm us with pure joy if we focus on them and allow them to.

Best Moments of the Day:

1. _____

2. _____

3. _____

Happiness is not an accident: Happiness is the result of changing your mentality, following your true purpose, and expressing genuine gratitude. It's a sign of satisfaction, a sign of achieving goals, and a sign of a fully functioning life. Happy people aren't just happy;

they've created their happiness. You can, too. It's easy! Easy, meaning something we can all do.

∽∽∽∽

Your thoughts and choices have immense power to raise your energy vibration, especially when you express gratitude. Each action that you take toward improving yourself will be reflected in the life you live, the prosperity you have, and the happiness that you feel. In the act of earnestly striving for improvement, the way will be cleared for you to experience a true peace within yourself. You will begin to find the answers you've been seeking.

You are the only one who will be with you forever, so make your experience with yourself as pleasant as you can by using the tools in this chapter to harness energy for your own benefit. Happiness is waiting for you. . . .

CHAPTER 7

Meditation:
Your Secret Superpower

I have experienced anxiety attacks for as long as I can remember. They would happen to me whenever I got incredibly upset about something (which was often). Suddenly, without warning, my breath would become shallow. When one, two, three breaths wouldn't come in fully, my eyes got wide. Instead of getting better, my breaths became shorter and shorter. Within seconds, dizziness started. Then, a tingling in my hands. Shivers up my spine. Icicles stinging my lungs. Small beads of perspiration on my forehead. Numbness in my face. Hiccups if I tried to speak.

When these panic attacks didn't go away after a moment, it threw me into sheer terror. Of course the terror made the attack even worse. Within a minute I was on my bed or the floor feeling like I'd been punched in the gut, was having the worst asthma attack of my life, and was drowning—all at the same time. At once a flood of emotions, memories, and helpless feelings coursed through me, and it took everything in me to not start hysterically crying, which I knew would only make it more difficult to breathe.

I didn't realize that these attacks were not "normal" until many years later, after a doctor diagnosed me with anxiety in high school. Medication was prescribed for it, but medication never treated it. I had not learned how to control the unhealthy, vicious cycle, so each time I felt a wave of strong emotion, I always panicked. It seemed like I could never gain control of my thoughts or my mind. I felt like a prisoner to my own body.

It took me many years, but I did finally find one tool that allowed me to conquer anxiety attacks completely. This tool not only alleviated the panic attacks but also has allowed me to conquer other forms of anxiety, such as social anxiety and my fear of heights and planes. It's brought success, health, and prosperity into my life, time and time again, and it's allowed me to manifest so many of my dearest goals. That tool is meditation, and it completely saved my life. It can save yours, too.

Why Meditation Works

Meditation is a discipline for training the mind to develop a clear and evocable calm, and then using that calm to bring a larger understanding to your life and the world. The greater your understanding of the world, the more freedom you will have in your life. The more freedom we have to live as we please, the more we feel confident in our ability to conduct our lives in a way that will bring us the greatest amount of peace, joy, wisdom, wealth, and health. Meditation is a way of slowing down so that we can easily get in touch with who we are. It helps us access our deep inner resource for healing, calming the mind, and operating more effectively in the world.

A study from the University of Wisconsin-Madison indicates that the practice of meditation reduces the grey matter density in areas of the brain related with anxiety and stress. Grey matter regions of the brain command important abilities and skills like muscle control, emotions, self-control, decision making, and sensory perceptions such as sight, memory, speech, and hearing. Meditators in the study were more able to "attend moment-to-moment to the stream of stimuli to which they are exposed and less likely to 'get stuck' on any one stimulus." The kind of meditation studied involves mindfulness: nonreactively monitoring the content of experience from moment-to-moment as a means to recognize the nature of emotional and cognitive patterns.[13] The study also noted that an eight-week meditation practice may be effective for reducing stress and increasing quality of life and self-compassion.

Stress, for example, has been clinically proven to worsen inflammation. Skin specialists have recorded that life's stress can cause flare-ups in inflammatory disorders such as psoriasis, acne, arthritis, and eczema. Yep—that's why you nearly *always* break out when you're stressed! Stress may affect inflammation in the skin, the joints, or the muscles. The larger indication is that this is part of an ancient biological response, a warning sign to our system. This might be one of the largest bodies of evidence that the body and mind are undoubtedly connected. Our bodies respond physically to emotional distress.

Jon Kabat-Zinn, Professor of Medicine Emeritus and creator of the Stress Reduction Clinic and the Center for Mindfulness in Medicine, Health Care, and Society at the University of Massachusetts Medical School, found compelling evidence that mind-strengthening techniques provide significant anti-inflammatory relief. It was clinically found that meditation and stress-control techniques can help to speed healing from psoriasis and other inflammatory skin conditions. Even novice meditators—those who practiced only thirty-five minutes per day at home—had smaller patches of inflammation compared to the control groups.[14]

We can only focus on one thought at a time. Try it—you'll see! Although at times your mind may seem to "race," really, you can only hold one thought at any given moment. When you focus on one thing, you are forced to ignore everything else. Whatever you focus on, your body naturally responds to. The more control you have of your thoughts, the more control you gain of your body. The more control that you have over your body, the more you can dominate your health, wellness, lifestyle, job, and start to really achieve—and then surpass—your dearest dreams and goals.

Your WILD Meditation Habit

In another research study published in the *American Journal of Psychiatry,* twenty-two patients diagnosed with anxiety disorder or panic disorder were submitted to three months of meditation and relaxation training. In just those three months, an impressively significant twenty of those twenty-two patients reported that the effects of their panic and anxiety had reduced substantially, and the changes were maintained at follow-up.[15]

Meditation is an unlocked superpower and we all come equipped with the ability to use it. We just need to learn how to tap into it.

Stress is a form of anxiety. The unknown is what gives you anxiety and stresses you out. Every time you feel anxious, you have to remember to make a conscious effort to relax. This is no simple task. The scary symptoms you may experience during anxiety attacks or stressful situations (such as shortness of breath, tingling, foggy thoughts, or numbness) all relate back to your heart rate. You want your heart rate to be as low as possible to overcome anxiety, and you'll definitely need it low in order to resist a full-blown panic attack. To do this, you absolutely need to train your body. The more you react calmly when your body screams emotional chaos, the easier it becomes to do. Soon enough, this reaction is natural. When you feel anxious, your body won't automatically release adrenaline and speed up your heart rate. Instead, it will release calming hormones and give you the space you need to think and overcome whatever challenges you encounter.

This is your new WILD habit overcoming your harmful habit.

Over time you will be able to instantly relax and quickly (but calmly) assess the situation you're in. *Are you in any real danger? Is there anything that can really hurt you right now? How can you deal with this in a positive way?* The answers to these kinds of questions become clear and automatic.

Belly breathing, one of the most essential tricks to successfully meditating, is the first step. Once you recognize what's truly going on, go straight into one of my favorite meditation practices:

- Take a deep breath into your diaphragm through your nose. Do this until your belly is completely swollen with air and then begin to hold your breath for four seconds, or four heartbeats.

- Release the breath through your mouth.

- Repeat.

- Once you can successfully fill your belly, release your breath on the count of five heartbeats.

- Repeat until you feel a sense of personal warmth and calm.

Practice this exercise every single day, no matter what. Find time first thing in the morning, during breaks throughout the day, and/or right before bed at night. Regardless of whether feeling overwhelmed has become our culture's new "normal," it's not normal, and it never should be. You can have a hundred things to do without becoming completely overwhelmed. You need to find the space to recognize exactly what's going on—and this starts in your mind. That's where meditation comes in! This simple practice gives you the time to understand why you are feeling overwhelmed and anxious. Within a few moments, you can prioritize what needs to be weighing on your heart. You can assess what is truly important, and you can let go of what you are holding on to unnecessarily.

The more you practice this, the easier it will become. Meditation hones our intuition and improves our clarity. Soon enough, it becomes a lifestyle. If your mind is focused on your stress, stress is what you will feel. When we give ourselves the space to focus elsewhere, we give ourselves an attitude of surrender. When we surrender in this way, we can think our way into whatever kind of body or life that we choose. Mindful meditation is step one.

Common Harmful Meditation Habits:

Becoming bored

Thinking it "doesn't apply to you" or "won't work for you"

Thinking your brain "races too fast" to practice meditation (this is exactly why you need to start!)

Believing your chronic pain or illness can prevent you from meditation (in fact, you can do it laying down or in any way that's comfortable for you)

Believing that you don't have the time

Giving yourself excuses to stop

Stopping your practice

WILD Meditation Habits:

Practicing meditation for at least 5 to 10 minutes every day

Working up to a longer period every time you practice (15 minutes, then 30 minutes, then 60 minutes)

Realizing that doing nothing IS doing something—you are training your body to relax

Reminding yourself of the health and wellness benefits you're giving yourself with this simple new habit

Embracing your new, secret superpower and allowing it to affect other areas of your life, such as your work or your family dynamic

Getting excited to meditate by giving yourself a "reward," like a banana cacao smoothie, after your practice

Becoming thrilled to meditate so that you can harness your thoughts and have control over your life

Mindful Meditation Rituals

Meditation is the simplest form of mind-work. Sitting quietly gives us the time and tools to learn truths about ourselves we'd *never* figure out otherwise. One of the first things I learned in meditation was that my normal breathing was totally panicked. Well, no wonder I had anxiety! I didn't need medication—I needed to figure out how to breathe!

Most of the harmful habits that hold us back from our dreams are learned behaviors that we may not even realize we have. It wasn't until I started meditating that things really began falling into place for me. When I got into a steady routine in my meditation practice, I was able to give up a lot of ego gratification, which left room for amazing things to manifest. Soon I was looking at a life full of new friendships, amazing opportunities, and fearless action. Without mind-work, you won't be able to find the strength needed to conquer learned helplessness, which becomes totally ingrained in us.

To make room for mind-work, you need to be consistent. Making a plan is the only way to do this at first. Without a plan there is no way a new habit—especially an often foreign one like meditation—can become ingrained into our daily lives over time. Practice meditation in the same way you practice any new habit: Repeat it at the same time every day. Plant your seed of meditation and water it day in and day out. There is hardly a pleasure greater than thinking nothing—that is why it's called pure bliss.

During meditation, there is no pressure to be anywhere but simply in the moment. Your practice is where you completely connect to your higher self, who carries no guilt and no ego. When you practice your meditation habit, your higher self becomes a stronger force. She can bestow the ultimate forgiveness to you, allowing you to let go of anything that no longer serves you.

Don't allow excuses like "I don't have the time" or "I can't concentrate" to sneak up on you. Without meditation, or without taking time to focus on what's really important, goals are lost, time is wasted, and nothing else matters! We live in a culture where we keep ourselves so constantly scheduled, and where we are so often connected to technology, that we rarely take the time to simply *be* and to think about life. You need to meditate every day, for at least five minutes a day. Period. While meditating take a moment to include love and gratitude for your body and its healing work. Take a silent few minutes to acknowledge any or all the things you're truly grateful for. Focus on happy highlights of the day and send prayers and thoughts to your loved ones for five minutes. You can gradually increase your time as you get used to it to fifteen minutes, thirty minutes, or even a full hour on certain days.

It can be incredibly difficult to focus and relax, so this is where repetition becomes paramount. Many people give up because they feel that they're too busy to meditate or they feel they can't slow down their thoughts. You may find that the more you try NOT to picture something, the more easily it shows up.

This is natural. It helps to overcome this by picturing a blank stage like at a movie theater or a theater show. Stare at this blank stage and focus on your breath. This is the stage of your life. If thoughts or images you're trying to solve pop up on your stage, go back to making the screen in your mind completely black. Focus on your breath once again. Always come back to your breath. Instead of taking one breath in and one breath out, take two rapid breaths in through your nose and let it out in one solid, relaxed breath when you exhale. Two breaths in, one calm breath out. You'll find that the more you picture a blank slate and focus on your breath, the easier it becomes to cure yourself of racing thoughts or your to-do list.

It won't happen the first time or overnight; that's why we call meditation a *practice.* You need to keep at it and begin to find ways to practice meditation in your everyday life instead of just on your meditation pillow or before you slip off to sleep. The more you practice, the more you strengthen your meditation habit. Since I first began my daily meditation practice, I also started incorporating more meditation into my day-to-day routine, which has really helped me to assess my priorities and focus on my goals without getting overwhelmed. Mindful meditation can be done anywhere, and it truly helps immediately!

One of my favorite mindful meditations only takes five minutes, and I do it every day. I light a stick of incense on my mantle, which contains photographs of my relatives—Christmas snaps, family photos, black-and-white pictures of my great-great-grandparents on their wedding days. For the five minutes while the incense burns, I say a prayer and perform a silent meditation, sending my family health and light. I literally picture a ball of light traveling from my heart, across a map of the country, into their homes and lighting them up. This practice seems to have worked wonders, as members of my family have found themselves visited less by sickness and health issues since I began this meditation practice seven years ago.

The effort to complete this small mindful ritual is minimal but the reward you'll receive for doing it is enormous. Once you begin to function on the vibrations of love, peace, tranquility, and clarity, you will begin to attract much more of the same. Meditation connects you to your body as well as your mind. This practice sets the stage for a much more manageable life.

Very often we fall into ruts in our lives. We maintain the same routines and act in the same way day after day. This forms some of our most destructive and harmful habits. Mindful meditation is as simple as it is effective, and it can break us out of these ruts. Meditation is your body's way of truly "escaping" the stress of the real world by bringing your mind back to center for a few moments and remembering what's truly important: the fact that you're breathing. And that means you're truly alive. If we go through life unthinking and unchanged, we cannot access our true power.

A Mindful Meditation: Your Dream Life

One of the most powerful mindful meditations is to picture your life as you'd truly like it to be. Here is how to practice it:

- Have a seat, with your feet firmly planted on the ground. Lay down comfortably if sitting is in any way uncomfortable. Close your eyes. Take a deep breath into your diaphragm through your nose.

- Do this until your belly is completely swollen with air and then release your breath through your mouth.

- Repeat your inhale through your nose and exhale through your mouth, smoothing your breath as you release it.

- Picture a blank, black stage in your mind. Once you can successfully picture the stage blank, picture the healthiest,

most attractive, most vibrant version of yourself on it.
Maybe you come out singing and dancing. Maybe you're
just strolling along slowly. But remember, it's just you
against a black background on a stage, like at a theater.

∽ Now fill the black background with light. The light over-
whelms everything at first and then gets dimmer until it
is just lighting you and the area around you. As you focus
on yourself, you now see on the stage that you are against
a background of your wildest dreams. Maybe it's you walking to your dream job in New York City or lounging on
the beach with your dogs in Hawaii. Maybe you're signing
autographs, accepting an Olympic Gold medal, or giving
birth to a healthy child. Whatever you picture as your best
life, see that as the background to you on the stage.

∽ Now someone emerges and asks you, "How did you get
here?"

∽ Feel free to take a moment, and then answer them.

∽ Take them back. Take them back to the beginning, through
the last few years or months or weeks, to how you accomplished your goal. Explain it in as much detail as possible.
Maybe you trained hard every day. Maybe you worked your
ass off with little payoff for a long time. Maybe terrible circumstances pushed you to find a better way to live. Perhaps
you simply fell in love. Whatever brought you to your dream
life, delve into it. Picture it in as much detail as you can;
elaborate on every step of the way.

∽ When you're finished explaining your route to success to
the person, allow the lights on stage to dim.

∽ They dim slowly until your stage is black again.

∽ Open your eyes.

This meditation should not only reveal your deepest desires but also the path to get there. Mindful meditation can help us to make the impossible in our life absolutely, truly, and miraculously possible. When you gain this control, you can begin to create a plan and a realistic pathway. Done earnestly every day without discouragement, this practice inevitably leads to success, which propels our inner peace.

Meditation for Pain

Researchers at Group Health Research Institute in Seattle recently found that they could cure lower back pain—with mindfulness meditation! The scientists randomly assigned 342 adults with chronic lower back pain to receive either two-hour weekly sessions of group meditation training or standard medical care (which could include options like physical therapy or painkillers). Six months later, the participants in the meditation group had an easier time climbing stairs, pulling on socks, and getting up out of a chair, and they were less likely to be bedridden than the other groups who received physical therapy and painkillers. Of patients in the meditation group, 60 percent showed a "meaningful" improvement in their daily activities. A year later and they were still doing better.[16]

If you're looking to eradicate the source of your pain, look no further. Whether you're fighting a disease that affects your whole body, or your pain is localized to one spot, try this meditation to help your body fight your pain in a natural, positive way.

- Sit with your feet firmly planted on the ground or lay down if sitting is uncomfortable. Take a deep breath into your diaphragm through your nose.

- Do this until your belly is completely swollen with air and then release the breath through your mouth.

- Repeat the process of inhaling through your nose into your diaphragm and out slowly through your mouth. Focus on smoothing your breath.

- Place your hand over the source of your discomfort. Truly feel where your pain is coming from. Even when we have pain throughout our whole bodies, often it is emanating from one spot or source.*

- Now, slowly move your hand away from the source of your discomfort so that your palm is just a few inches from your body. Feel the heat of your body next to your hand. Focus on your hand's connection to your body—even though they are not touching, your body is aware of your hand and your hand is aware that it is close to your body.

- Feel your hand pulling the source of discomfort out of your body. Feel the pain rising as heat from your body and eliminating it into the atmosphere. Do this until you can truly *feel* your hand pulling this discomfort away.

- You will feel the discomfort diminish as you do so. As the pain diminishes, pull your hand farther and farther from your body.

- When you have successfully eliminated your uncomfortable feeling, even for a few moments, you may open your eyes.

- Repeat this meditation twice a day until your discomfort is gone.

This exercise not only helps us to identify the source of our discomfort but also trains our minds to dismantle and remove toxicity from our bodies. This increases our conscious awareness of our own

---

* If you can't reach the source of your pain, practice this exercise in your mind's eye, simply imagining it happening with your eyes closed.

personal dis-ease and brings comfort and true healing. We are not just picturing our pain melting away—we are truly *practicing* melting our pain away with this incredible self-healing technique.

Meditation for Mental Distress

Once I started meditating in 2011, anxiety was one of the first afflictions I was almost immediately able to control. In just a few short weeks, any time I encountered stress, I was somehow able to take a breath and successfully relax. It was no small miracle!

You can train your brain to remain calm and look at life from a more positive, relaxed perspective this way. In fact, it's the most simple and effective tool. Our minds can only focus on one thing at a time. We must choose what to focus on.

Focus on concentration of breath for a peaceful life. As the breath flows, so flows the mind, because there is a feedback system between the mind and the breath. As the breath becomes calmer, so does the mind, and vice versa. The more you concentrate on your breath, the quieter your mind becomes.

Right now, pharmaceutical medication is the most common treatment for those suffering from ADHD (attention deficit hyperactivity disorder), the off-the-cuff diagnosis I had received as a teenager. I'm certainly not alone. Roughly 11 percent of children have been diagnosed with ADHD in their lifetime. However, it looks as though mindfulness meditation has a more significant impact on those suffering from ADHD than medication. A study conducted in 2013 by the *Journal of Attention Disorders* on mindfulness meditation training in adults with ADHD was intensely promising. Rigorous testing and repeated assessments were done on two groups diagnosed with ADHD and taking medication: One group received mindfulness meditation training and one group did not. To evaluate the impact of mindfulness training, multiple measures were collected from the participants who meditated and control participants before treatment began, during several days in the eight-week program, and immediately after treatment ended. The results were dramatic.

Compared to control participants, adults who received mindfulness meditation training reported statistically significant and clinically meaningful declines in core ADHD symptoms, both inattentive symptoms and hyperactive-impulsive symptoms. Nearly 64 percent of adults receiving meditation treatment reported at least a 30 percent decline in their symptoms, compared to a whopping 0 percent in the control group. Participants felt the mindfulness meditations were easy to integrate into their lifestyle. The group who meditated attended nearly 90 percent of scheduled sessions and the average treatment satisfaction rating was 5.91 on a 7 point scale, reflecting a very high degree of satisfaction. Meditation participants reported significant gains in their ability to regulate emotions and tolerate distress. Almost all the meditation participants felt confident that they would continue to use the techniques they had been taught well after the study ended.[17]

Meditation and Neuroplasticity

If we can use meditation as a powerful way to cure our pain, relax, fight the symptoms of an attention disorder, set our intentions, and accomplish our goals, *what else can it be used for?* Well, it turns out those who meditate may have created for themselves a built-in way to fight deadly illness.

In a study with Tibetan Buddhist monks conducted by neuroscientist Richard Davidson of the University of Wisconsin, it was found that novice meditators "showed a slight increase in gamma activity" but that most Tibetan monks showed "extremely large increases of a sort that has never been reported before in the neuroscience literature." Gamma rays can kill living cells, a fact which medicine uses to its advantage, using Gamma rays to kill cancerous cells as a form of high-energy radiation chemotherapy. It seems as though through their earnest daily meditation practice, these monks have given themselves the ability to fight cancer and other chronic diseases by naturally building up their gamma activity, without the use of aggressive Western medicine. For his discoveries on how meditation can positively affect the human brain, *Time Magazine* named Davidson one of the 100 Most Influential People in the World.[18]

Neuroplasticity is a term that is used to describe the brain changes that occur in response to experience. There are many different mechanisms of neuroplasticity, ranging from the growth of new brain connections to the creation of new neurons. When the framework of neuroplasticity is applied to meditation, the mental training of meditation is fundamentally no different than rewiring the brain. The essence of meditation is cultivating a greater awareness of what it means to be human, therefore making our problems easier to recognize and solve. There are very few people who couldn't benefit from a greater sense of awareness. If we learn how to become more in touch with the present moment, we automatically feel more vibrant, healthy, and alive.

Meditation empowers you. It deepens the value you place on your body, it enriches your day-to-day experiences, and it connects you with who you truly are. This ancient practice helps us to remember things we barely think about *at all* otherwise: how to breathe, how to manifest our destiny, and how to encourage our bodies to fight disease and obtain optimal health. Meditation becomes so deeply compelling that you don't ever want to stop once you see the incredible positive effects it has on your life. Why would you ever quit something that can benefit you so deeply? Why would you stop doing the one practice that can answer so many of life's unanswerable questions, like where the secret to health truly lies or how to calm our mind and control our thoughts? You wouldn't. You'd save yourself the grief of living the mundane, unfulfilling, and frustrating life that so many people are used to. The practice of meditation makes it clear what's in your best interest. If you start to understand what's in your own best interest, you can easily take your health into your own hands.

The Advantages of Meditation

Meditation can help us in so many areas of our lives. As our awareness increases, so does our ability to fight unwanted thoughts, infections, dis-ease, and illness. We can access the willpower necessary to take control of our lives. This is transcendence—transcendence from fear, transcendence from illness, and freedom from mental slavery. Once you have this transcendence, you've reached a plane of enlightenment.

We can use the WILD Method to help us commit to our practice. We must be *willing* to let go of our preconceived notions about meditation and use our *intuition* to discern how a meditation practice can enrich our lives. Then we must show the *love* that it takes to carve out time for ourselves to make our practice a daily ritual and a new WILD habit. Finally, we need to keep up the *discipline* it takes for meditation to have a lasting, long-term positive effect on our whole lives.

What Are Your Meditation Advantages?

List the advantages of getting started in your meditation practice today. Here are some examples:

Examples of meditation advantages:

1. I will feel proud of myself if I get started.

2. I'll be able to think more clearly and feel more in control.

3. I am on my way to becoming someone who is healthier, happier, and has less stress in my life.

4. My significant other and family will be pleasantly surprised.

Advantages of my mediation practice:

1. _____

2. _____

3. _____

4. _____

Truly think about all of the advantages there are to beginning a meditation practice today; they far outweigh any disadvantages of possibly feeling uncomfortable or like a novice (feelings that really only pop up the very first time anyway). The more you practice, the easier it becomes. You may experience an instant lift in your mood, a newfound self-respect, or higher self-esteem. Like many who make an earnest start, you'll see a significant improvement in your health and wellness in no time at all. If you're one of the lucky few who makes this practice a daily part of your life, you may get to sit back and watch your dearest goals and dreams begin to manifest, as you apply the meditations and mind-strengthening techniques laid out in this book.

Think of meditation as an advantage you have in life. Most other people have no tools handy to solve their issues (because really, who *does* practice meditation every day?!). Unfortunately, the majority of the world misses out. This places you in a small percentage of people who are connected to the universe in a personal, scientific, sacred, and natural way. Meditation is truly your secret superpower. It's a valuable asset. Would you rather be the authority on Stressing Out or Zen-ing Out? Meditation is a serious nonnegotiable for achieving a better life.

PART 3

WILD BODY

CHAPTER 8

The Good Food and Exercise Habit

I used to wake up with a feeling of complete dread every day, as I continually faced an unsatisfying, uphill, and depressing New York City lifestyle that seemed impossible to escape. A typical weekday in my early twenties would have found me struggling to get up around dawn, scrambling to find clean work clothes, and racing to make the first of half a dozen buses, trains, and subways I took to work at a listless job that neither excited nor inspired me.

I had a corporate and scientific resume—neither of which reflected my true dreams or goals. I was barely eating, hardly sleeping, and I was desperately addicted to my prescription drugs to solve my pain, problems, and personality. Every day for eleven years I woke up, got dressed, filled a glass of cloudy tap water, and took a handful of pills. I would then try to eat something dairy and carb heavy right before school or on my way to my job. If I was lucky, I ate lunch many hours later, and it consisted of whatever I could afford (which, for the record, was not much). Dinner usually came in a greasy paper bag. The dollar menu was my BFF.

I was popping around fourteen different kinds of medications all day long, adding up to a nauseating amount of pills. This was, in one way or another, intended to attack the kind of pain that hits you and can't be explained with words. It's an empty pain that crushes the heart and lives in the stomach. Debilitating, all-encompassing, body-bruising pain that carries heaviness in your chest. Whether it's caused by crushing anxiety, accidental injury, seemingly inborn depression, or survivor's guilt, it's the kind of pain that seduces you to reach for a bottle of pills, even though they never work, just for some semblance of relief. Maybe today, just once, you think, they will actually *do* something.

So at night I'd knock myself out on a muscle relaxer or a sleeping pill or a tall glass of booze, and I would say a silent prayer that the emptiness would be gone tomorrow, or at least a little dulled, so that maybe I could cope.

Food was the last thing on my mind.

Today, food is paramount in my life. Nutrition was the key that unlocked my personal health and wellness, and I've seen it change so many thousands of people's lives for the better firsthand.

My WILD Food Habits

Today, I wake up in the morning and the first thing I do is hydrate. Ice water with a slice of organic, hand-picked lemon to balance my skin and detoxify me, caffeine-free, herbal tea made of anti-inflammatory herbs, and kombucha—a probiotic beverage that protects my gut health—are first on the list. I will then make a veggie or fruit smoothie and take my supplements. If I feel like my blood sugar is high, I make a green smoothie; if I feel that it's low, I make a fruit smoothie. This is all before I start to cook a high-protein breakfast: oatmeal, poached eggs, an organic baked potato, raw avocado, and sometimes a protein like chicken on a bed of greens. While this may be a heavy breakfast for some, I am normally extremely hungry in the morning, and it works optimally for me.

I need this kind of protein-rich meal in the morning, since one of the first activities of my day is to take my two rescued pit bull mixes, Raelie and Ruca, on a hike. Whether we hike through the local Torrey Pines or throw the ball around on the dog beach, it's important for me to get my blood flowing first thing in the morning. Otherwise, I start to feel stagnant and pain creeps in.

For lunch, I'll make myself another meal from scratch: rice or quinoa with a protein like tofu or meat, and veggies. I can turn this into a bowl, a salad, or a gluten-free sandwich. The possibilities are endless.

I snack a lot, but in tiny portions. I snack about once an hour throughout the day, which I realize is probably not the best advice for everyone, but it's honestly what works for me and keeps me stabilized and not hangry (hungry + angry). I go for healthy snacks like fruit salad, coconut chips, or gluten-free pretzels with almond butter. I avoid sugar and processed foods and replace table salt with Himalayan sea salt.

I keep my meals fresh, bright, and light. Dinner comes after another sundown hike with the dogs and is the most exciting meal for me to cook, since I am more freed up from work and not as much of a slave to my blood sugar by dinnertime. I can make a strawberry and arugula salad, cook up some crab and artichokes, or make polenta encrusted salmon. Desserts are now healthy versions of what I used to enjoy: sugar-free coconut ice cream, dairy-free dark chocolate, or almonds drizzled with organic honey.

I only eat out a handful of times a year, mostly for social events and while I'm traveling. This helps a lot. I'm not a slave to other people's nutritional choices, and I don't have to worry about how my food was cooked. I no longer give into cravings that I can recognize are triggered by outside circumstances, events, or even my favorite TV show. Sometimes the activities we engage in or the shows we watch will trigger us to crave certain foods, for instance if we ate those same foods the last time we heard that theme song or recognized that actor's voice. Pavlov proved this in his famous experiments with dogs: Every time Pavlov fed his dogs, he rang a bell. He repeated this experiment until the dogs associated hearing the bell with eating their food. Then Pavlov rang a bell and served no food. The dogs still salivated and acted like their food was on its way. They salivated every time they heard the bell, food or no food. We have this exact same conditioning process.

I have no reservations about food and often others have poked fun at me because I certainly don't look like I eat basically every hour that I'm awake (thank you, metabolism and exercise). But I will never take the privilege of having healthy food around me lightly. After more than twenty-five years of living off two hundred dollars a month in food stamps and almost three years of constant nausea from withdrawal, I'll never again take my nutrition for granted.

Food vs. Antidepressants

Did you know that there is no scientific link between serotonin level and depression? That's right, depression is not merely a "chemical imbalance," as we're so often led to believe. Researchers admittedly still don't understand all the causes of depression. In fact, no scientific or laboratory test of any kind exists that can even test for or confirm that someone truly *has* a mental illness!

First, let's tackle the idea of the "chemical imbalance" that underlies the serotonin theory of depression. In order for us to suggest an imbalance in your brain, first we'd have to understand what a perfectly balanced brain looks like. To date, no study or researcher has been able to show such a brain. It simply doesn't exist. The brain is the least-understood organ in the body today. What we do know about it is that it is constantly changing and virtually any stimuli from any of our senses is able to alter it temporarily. We don't understand why the brain is structured the way it is, or even how it actually communicates internally (although we have a lot of working theories).

An analysis of over 14,000 patients with mental illness was conducted by Dr. Thomas Insel, former head of The National Institute of Mental Health (NIMH.) He admitted, "Despite high expectations, neither genomics nor imaging has yet impacted the diagnosis or treatment of the 45 million Americans with serious or moderate mental illness each year." This means that despite there being 45 million Americans who suffer from mental illness every year, there is absolutely no test out there that exists that can identify and locate mental illness in the body. You can't give someone a blood test and diagnose them with bipolar disorder. You can't take a scan of the body and say definitively that someone has anxiety. You can't graph mental illness, you can't measure it, and you can't pull it up on an MRI. Doctors rely simply on questions and answers for diagnosing their patients. The problem with this method is that it's subject to human error and, therefore, not always accurate. What if you misunderstood a question or two? What if you're in a bad mood? What if the doctor has a bias toward someone who looks like you, therefore diagnosing you incorrectly based on his or her own precognition?

Your doctor then takes these answers you provide and checks them against his or her DSM and psychiatric knowledge, which also might be inaccurate, out of date, or predisposed to bias. Diagnosing mental illness with the classic question-and-answer method leaves a lot of room for error, but currently that is our most practiced and accepted method.

What is eye opening is that many common foods and spices, such as turmeric, have been proven to work *better* than common antidepressants like Prozac at treating depression in scientific studies. During a turmeric versus Prozac study, researchers found that those taking only Prozac improved 64.7 percent but suffered side effects. Those taking only turmeric improved 62.5 percent but suffered no side effects. Those taking a combination of both improved by a significant 77.8 percent.

The most concerning side effects of Prozac and other antidepressants on the market are suicidal thoughts, hallucinations, anxiety, and panic—the *exact* symptoms those who take the drug are looking to avoid. Turmeric, however, does not have any side effects. Unlike Prozac, turmeric is effective and safe when it comes to the treatment of depression. Frightening side effects present in patients who take Prozac are clearly absent in turmeric use.

Researchers noted: "This study provides first clinical evidence that turmeric may be used as an effective and safe modality for treatment in patients with major depressive disorder without concurrent suicidal ideation or other psychotic disorders."[19]

This is because nature encourages our bodies to be in balance, while pills deliver us chemicals and hope for the best.

The Power of Food

Food isn't merely food. Food is energy. Food is survival. Food is what builds and repairs. Food is both health and medicine. What you allow into your body, you become. I don't prescribe or subscribe to a certain label or diet. I believe in listening to what your body is telling you about food.

If you're craving chocolate, for example, that's your body giving you a message. Perhaps the message is low blood sugar or a magnesium deficiency. Perhaps, though, *The Bachelor* just started, and you always eat chocolate while watching *The Bachelor*. Here is how you can practice a quick mental assessment to see what your body needs versus what you're craving:

1. *What is happening in my environment right now?* Are you stressed out or happy? This is where you might notice that *The Bachelor* is on and start to go back to the last time you were in this place. Take a quick look around and assess your surroundings as well as your mental state.

2. *Am I truly hungry?* Are you being stimulated by your surroundings (such as the theme song to *The Bachelor*) or are you really, *truly* hungry? Are you dealing with a breakup and this is a way to cope? If your belly isn't growling and gurgling, the answer is probably no, you're not *truly* hungry. If the answer is yes, move on to question #3.

3. *Is there anything healthier that I can enjoy or do to satisfy my cravings?* Can you go for a leisurely hike or a walk around the block? Can you meditate on your harmful habits? Can you choose a different food that still satisfies your chocolate cravings, like an organic cacao and almond milk smoothie?*

Food should have little to do with a number on a scale. Some people, such as those who body build or struggle with weight issues, are actually attempting to gain weight when they eat. Always ask yourself *why* you're eating what you're eating. Do a quick mental assessment about how much food you eat to satisfy cravings and how much food you eat to propel your goals forward. Find what your body needs instead of what you've trained yourself to crave. To have a new life, you need to truly let go of everything that led to your old life.

Instead of seeing failure as a setback, let it inspire you to do better next time. Think of it this way: now you know what NOT to do. After only a short while, it becomes clear that indulging in old, harmful

---

* Combine one teaspoon raw organic cacao and one cup of coconut or almond milk into a blender. Blend on high. You can also use the same ingredients and add them to a cup of hot water for a little organic hot cocoa. *So* delicious. Enjoy!

habits begins to disrespect and undermine all of the hard work you've done on yourself! There are small tweaks you can make to turn around your harmful body habits and replace them with WILD habits. If you crave sugar, eat fruits. If you want to lose weight, drink more water when you feel cravings. Any time you are deciding what to eat, when to eat, or how to eat, use the WILD Method:

- Be *Willing* to listen to your body. Are you eating from hunger or boredom? If your only food choice is carrot sticks (and not potato chips), would you still eat them?

- Have the *Intuition* to process and understand your body's true needs. Are you eating what your body is truly craving or did you grab something else? Maybe you picked up a blueberry muffin but your body actually *needed* a blueberry and coconut milk smoothie. Take a quick mental assessment and be honest with yourself.

- Be *Loving* in your approach to what you choose to feed your body. Treat your body like it is the most precious thing you have (because it is!). Give it the vitamins and minerals in leafy greens and veggies, not chemical-laden fast or processed food.

- Ask yourself if your choice aligns with your *Discipline*. For instance, will eating a salad help you move toward your goal better than any other nutritional choice?

The X Factor

Depression, anxiety, and mental illness are real, and they all contribute to our body image. I know that because I've experienced them all. I've suffered from low self-esteem, I've been a victim of bullying about my looks and weight, and I've been at the precipice of ending my own life. I would never deny that medication has saved many people's lives, I just don't think it solves the whole equation—not for our body, mind, spirit, or healing process. Medication is not "X." Medication can be part of the equation that eventually leads to "X."

Think of it this way:

$$\text{Medication} + \text{Good Nutrition} + \text{Meditation} +$$
$$\text{20 Mins of Exercise/Day} = X$$

$$X = \text{A better life!}$$

"X" is your goal. It can be whatever you want. X can be: Run a marathon this summer! X can be: Have a better relationship with my spouse. This is your personal X Factor. Think about this as you are building your dream self and replacing harmful habits with WILD habits.

Maybe medication needs to be a part of your daily routine— maybe it doesn't. In whatever way you are choosing to treat your body, remember that balance is the key. If you are going to take anti-anxiety medication, remember to work toward addressing the cause of your anxieties. Have you been spending enough time focused on your goals? Are you checking things off your to-do list? Are you possibly contributing to your own stress somehow? Can incorporating meditation or a brisk walk into your daily routine work in tandem with your medication to help you learn another way to remain calm during times of stress?

It won't be one or two things that add up to a more balanced existence. It will be a few simple moves every day that really make the difference and create a unique synergy together that improves your life. Self-love begins here.

Finding Balance in Your Habits

Our personal habits are the most important actions we can take toward improvement. Be mindful about your movement, your food habits, and your fitness. Be careful about the kind of thoughts you allow into your consciousness. Keep negative self-talk OUT.

Stand guard at the door to your mind. Do not allow any thoughts in that do not serve you or propel your life. Leave room for all the good stuff: self-love, care, and positive energy. You know the right path or purpose for you. We all have that inner voice of intuition that knows when to stop and how to improve. We need to tune in and listen to it.

The second you begin thinking about something bad, find a thought or a goal to replace it with. For instance, if you keep harping on an argument with your mother, think to yourself that you will instead work on good thoughts that will propel or stabilize your relationship with her, instead of allowing yourself to let anger or negativity take over. This is the way to simultaneously control our thoughts and address our problems head on. We're not trying to make harmful habits go away immediately: We're trying to solve their root cause so that they naturally disappear on their own.

Without the correct personal habits, it's hard for the body to do *anything* to its full potential. It's difficult to process emotions, to think correctly, or to make good decisions. These are the habits that affect our body the most, such as choosing what to eat, when to eat, how to exercise, when to move, when to meditate, and so on.

When we're neglecting our personal habits, we're neglecting ourselves. For instance, I was neglecting my personal habits and myself when I was relying on pills to solve my problems instead of giving holistic health and fitness the necessary place in my life to truly change me for good.

Mindful Nutrition

A diet is nutritionally defined as the kind of food that a person habitually eats. It can be for medical reasons or personal goals, and it usually varies from person to person. I don't believe that there is *one* plan or one diet out there that will work for absolutely everyone. Epigenetics proves this. The environmental effect to our genes is often unknown until after the effects have begun to show. For instance, an identical set of twins may eat the exact same food, but due to separate exercise patterns, environmental factors, or metabolism, their weight may be different or distributed in completely separate areas.

Why is this? There is a certain predisposition involved, but for the most part, only *we* affect our physical outcome. We may be predisposed to certain tendencies, but we are the only ones making the choices about what to put into our body, how often to move, where to live, how much exercise to get, and so on.

As individuals, we come with our own personal strengths, deficiencies, and unique nutritional needs. When we unlock what those are for us personally, we can take control of our so-called "diets," notice our patterns, break our bad behaviors, and ultimately transform our lives. I've done this with great success, and I've taught and observed many other people do it with amazing results as well.

I've watched women who battled weight issues their entire life finally decide to run a 5K (and do it!). I've witnessed frustrated young ladies who struggled with body image issues for years completely overcome their self-destructive tendencies and find true nourishment and happiness. I've seen countless men who worked their way to a new body and gave themselves a second chance, after a devastating loss or divorce. And I've observed beautiful mothers who thought they'd "never lose the baby weight" now proudly model for lingerie companies! All because they recognized their harmful habits, tapped into their intuition, asked themselves the right questions, and accessed their personal power. They started practicing WILD habits, overcoming what may otherwise have become lifelong struggles against themselves.

What we eat isn't about dieting. A diet is a plan on a piece of paper. Eating is about nourishment. Eating is about joy. Eating is about balance. It's time we shift our internal conversation from food to nutrition. I have noticed a distinct trend in my own personal nutritional journey and those of my friends and family after making this mental transition. Unlocking the key to our particular perfect nutritional habits and, moreover, our perfect life lies in our body habits.

You'll know what's healthy for you to eat because you'll *feel good* when you eat it. Not bloated, full, or gross. You'll be pleasantly full. You'll have energy you didn't know you had. Your skin will glow.

Doing the work doesn't mean depriving yourself, starving yourself, or being hard on yourself. Doing the work is about being *honest* with yourself. For example, maybe you love bagels, but they don't make you feel great when you eat them, and they make it harder for you to reach your ideal, healthy-for-you weight. However, when you start your day with scrambled eggs with lots of veggies, you feel incredible energy and focus better on your work. Doing the work of mindful eating isn't always easy, but it's always worth it. When you make food, fully engage in the activity. Smell your food before you cut or cook it—and smell it *after!* Use each one of your five senses any time you can. When you eat, ask yourself WHY you're eating everything you're eating.

Ask yourself what your ideal body looks like, what your specific weight goal is, and what you want your abs to look like—EXACTLY. Not what fifty different people who aren't you look like. If you can, try to use a photo of *yourself* at an ideal weight, shape, or size. One inspirational photo can keep you on track.

These three questions will keep you moving forward with your fitness goals:

1. Am I choosing to consume healthy foods every day? Why or why not?

2. Am I choosing to exercise every day? Why or why not?

3. How can I use better food choices and exercise to become a healthier person?

It all starts with your mind. Mind-strengthening techniques are the basis for change—especially nutritional change, which starts with your self-esteem. These techniques play a huge role in creating identity, progressive health patterns, personal success stories, and opportunities that will come your way. There is an art to manifesting and maintaining your health, improving your body, and achieving all of your goals and dreams. It starts with giving yourself the time to figure out what you really want—from your body and from your health. Even five minutes a day will do wonders for you.

You will never stick with a nutritional plan unless you put in the mind-work first. Apply the WILD Method to help you with your good food habits:

- Have the *Willingness* to change your habits.

- Use your *Intuition* to recognize which harmful food habits are holding you back.

- *Love* and accept yourself as you are at this present moment.

- Remain *Disciplined* so that you can picture a better future and continue to take the steps to reach it.

Often with nutrition, we can see results in mere hours. Getting the correct foods or supplements into our body—ones we may have been lacking our entire lives—can truly transform us. These foods can clear our skin, heal our gut, boost our brain, or give us renewed energy or a good night's sleep, literally overnight. Plants and people work in much the same way. Say you plant two identical pea plants right next to each other. These baby pea plants are in the same soil and exposed to the same sunlight. But if you spray organic nutrients on one plant's leaves and do not spray organic nutrients on the other plant's leaves, the plant that receives the nutrients will always grow bigger, taller, and stronger. Every single time. We also need the right kind of nutrients to become our best selves.

Today there are between 2.4 and 3.5 million annual physicians' visits for IBS (irritable bowel syndrome) in the US alone. Millions of people suffer from this condition, which affects the gut for unknown reasons. This may present as an upset stomach, cramping, change in bowel habits, abdomen pain, indigestion, or nausea. Maybe you've had these issues for years, but no doctor has ever been able to give you any solution that cured it. You can begin to help yourself by asking yourself questions about your dietary habits and willingness to change by using the WILD Method in order to promote self-healing:

1. What am I *Willing* to do to feel better? Are you willing to go out of your comfort zone to explore and incorporate natural methods to feel good?

2. Using your *Intuition,* ask yourself: Is there anything natural or healthy that I can take instead that will heal me? Through this question you may learn that, in fact, there are many ways to incorporate high-fiber, fermented, and probiotic foods into your diet, which can quickly heal and balance gut health. Stress and anxiety management also helps heal IBS.

3. Be *Loving* to yourself by cutting out anything that may be damaging to your gut health, like fried or processed foods, table salt, sugar, or alcohol. Make these observations without blame—as if you were watching a movie about someone else's life.

4. Be *Disciplined* in the actions you decide to take, and make your commitment long-term. That is truly the only way to see lasting benefits in your life.

The questions you ask yourself may lead you to admit to yourself that, *okay, maybe that glass of beer every night isn't helping to balance my body.* And, yes, maybe indulging in a salt fest or a sugar high more than three times a week is a big contributor to your digestive health, too. But because you've chosen to love yourself, without blame, you can make better decisions in the future. And you've already discovered what those decisions are: finding healthy, natural alternatives that support your gut health. This leads you to eating more fermented foods like kimchi and drinking more fermented, probiotic beverages such as kombucha. You begin to incorporate a probiotic supplement into your life every day, and along with your commitment to cutting out alcohol, sugar, and replacing table salt with Himalayan sea salt (which contributes to lower cholesterol), you start to feel much, much better. You meditate on a better version of your life—one without pain or a restrictive lifestyle. One day, you finally wake up without discomfort. From then on out, you *know* that you can live an untroubled, enjoyable life without digestive issues. A chronic problem that you dealt with for years can be there one day and gone the next—if you allow your WILD habits to take center stage and reboot your life.

Even if you're taking medication for treatment, you should be incorporating natural methods of healing into your everyday life.

The reason it's important to have go-to rituals and natural tools for healing is because at the end of the day, you can't rely on a pill. A pill won't do the work. You need to do the work. You need to be able to rely on yourself, no matter what. Correct nutritional habits make it much easier to rely on ourselves.

The Mindset Meditation

- Sit or lay in a comfortable position and close your eyes.
- Take a deep breath through your nose into your diaphragm, with your abdomen extended. Release your breath.
- Picture yourself at your ideal weight, shape, and size. Hold this image of yourself in your mind throughout your meditation. Breathe in, holding onto this image.
- Picture your ideal self doing the tasks it would take to get to that weight, shape, and size. See yourself waking up early and going on a run or making a healthy meal, dicing up vegetables on a chopping block. Breathe out, holding onto this image.
- Repeat these images for at least seven minutes a day without interruption.

This simple Mindset Meditation will put you in the correct mental space to begin the journey to a healthier life.

Natural Food Remedies

You get a sugar high. Then you crash. Then you crave something salty. Then you desire something sweet again. Your entire life revolves around this delicate balance, which never seems to be satisfied. Does this sound familiar? This is the nutritional roller coaster that most people are on. If we can get off of that roller coaster, we can dramatically improve our health.

To put the brakes on, we need to eat more vegetables, nuts, berries, fruit, and high-quality protein, at least once a week. Try incorporating sustainable, fresh, wild-caught seafood into your meal choices once a week. This will increase nutrient density—that means you'll obtain more of the vitamins, minerals, and essential fats that your body needs to thrive. Instead of indulging in something sugary, raise your vibration and level up on your choices, giving your body the foods it really needs for energy and healing.

I think a lot of people assume I'm vegan. I transitioned to raw food and veganism when I first changed my lifestyle, and I loved it. My body loved it at first, as it allowed me to basically "start over." It was simple—I only hit one or two aisles in the grocery store or took a leisurely stroll through the farmer's market and I was done. It vibes with my morals, my ideals, and my lifestyle. Veganism helps the planet, heals certain ailments, and has some of the most compassionate, inspired people in its community. I loved veganism, but unfortunately, over time, my body did not.

I had low energy and was constantly tired. My frame looked unhealthy. No matter how much I ate, I was constantly hungry. No meal ever seemed to completely satisfy my appetite. My skin was pale and my eyes were sunken in. I saw my doctor and had a blood test done. She explained that the results showed that my white blood cell count was incredibly low. I had severe anemia. Despite the fact that I was religiously eating vegan protein, my body didn't seem to be converting any of it to iron, a mineral we desperately need to regulate our blood and be healthy.

My doctor gave me two choices: a blood transfusion or a lifestyle change. She told me that even the blood transfusion would be a temporary fix. I'd never truly get better—if I didn't start eating meat. She said that without it I was bound to suffer from osteoarthritis, a painful arthritis of your bones.

I agonized a bit over this lifestyle change, wondering how I was EVER going to bring myself to buy or cook meat when I could not even walk down that aisle in the grocery store without being totally grossed out. This would be a complete 180 for me: a total switch in mentality and diet as well as a significant lifestyle change.

That same day, I assessed my *willingness* to change. Was I ready to start this process? Would it really have an impact? I knew in my heart that it would likely have a great benefit for me, but I needed some motivation, a way to rid myself of the guilt I currently felt associated with consuming meat.

I went into my nightly meditation practice and when I was done, I felt inspired to play a track from the great philosopher Alan Watts. My *intuition* led me to a live recording from his lectures in the 1960s. I hadn't listened to this track in many years, but a voice inside told me to take self-*loving* action and give myself a moment to absorb what Watts had to say. I used my *discipline* to simply sit and listen, hoping that the words would provide some clarity.

About a minute into the track, it hit me with goosebumps and chills. Here is what Alan Watts had told his students more than fifty years ago: "I challenged R. H. Blyth [an English author and famous vegetarian] and said, 'You're a vegetarian, but don't you realize that plants have feelings?' He said, 'Yes I do. . . . But they don't scream so loudly.'"

I realized that my own feelings toward life extended not just to the animals I might consume, but to everything that I consumed. I felt for the plants I ate almost in the same way I felt for the animals I ate, except the plants looked prettier, dressed up in wicker baskets at the farmer's market. As Blyth had so plainly said, they simply didn't scream as loud. I may be a sensitive person, but I couldn't very well *go on not eating what was good for my body*. I had to get over it. With this mental switch, I began to focus on what was best for my health.

I took my doctor's advice and started to buy grass-fed, organic meat. I had a very, very hard time cooking it, but also had an incredible support system around me who were encouraging my healthy actions. Honestly, once I began incorporating some chicken into my strawberry salad or some steak into my veggie sandwich, I saw a noticeable change in a very short amount of time. In just a few weeks, my energy levels were greatly improved, my skin glowed, I put on healthy weight, I found it easier to exercise, and I wasn't *constantly* hungry anymore. Ever since I started eating meat again, I truly began to feel like the real me. I understand the environmental, health, and moral consequences of eating meat, and that's why I encourage anyone who decides to consume meat to buy exclusively free-range, humanely-raised, hormone-free, organic meats. To offset the environmental impact of eating meat, I am personally an activist for many different animal rights causes. I'm an ambassador for the Lonely Whale Foundation and make yearly visits to organic, free-range farms. I've adopted all of my animals, and I eat exclusively grass-fed, organic, GMO-free meat. In fact, the same goes for any food: Buy organic, whenever possible. This might not be the right lifestyle for everyone, but I do believe we should all listen to our body. Plain and simple, I know I feel better.

Organic food may have higher nutritional value than conventional food, according to some research. That's because organic food has been grown and harvested without pesticides, chemicals, fertilizers, or GMOs, boosting the plant's production of vitamins and antioxidants that strengthen them and, in turn, strengthen *you* when you consume them. A study conducted by the National Academy of Science has linked pesticides in our food to everything from headaches to fertility issues to cancer and birth defects. This study suggests that even low-level pesticides can be significantly more toxic than organic food to pregnant women, fetuses, and babies, due to their less-developed immune systems, thereby putting an added tax on their organs. Organic meat is important because the antibiotics and growth hormones given to most farm animals can make our bodies resistant to drugs and more susceptible to bacteria that can harm us. You are what you eat: If the animals you consume have been fed growth hormones, antibiotics, or been kept in unsanitary conditions, you are exposing yourself and your body to those toxins and that energy.

Organic farming, on the other hand, reduces pollution in groundwater and creates richer soil for future plant growth. It also decreases the use of toxins that can wind up in your drinking water. Organic food has the highest vibration of any food because it has not been exposed to toxins. It is the way food is meant to be: simple, raw, and pure. Nutrition that's worry-free.

Kick the Cravings

Craving a candy bar? STOP. Do not pass GO and do NOT collect diabetes! Grab a handful of pomegranate seeds, a few squares of watermelon, or make a fruit smoothie! Make sure you reach for fruits over sweets. This will help you deal with your sugar cravings by satisfying your sweet tooth.

Raw, dark chocolate contains magnesium, which is nature's best chill pill, as well as essential fibers and B vitamins. But do not grab just any chocolate bar. Combine a small square of organic, raw dark chocolate that's dairy and sugar-free with a banana, a cup of strawberries, or a peach. You can even melt the chocolate and drizzle it over the fruit if that helps! Or blend some organic, raw cacao powder with a frozen banana and some coconut milk.

Grapes are also great for curbing your sweet tooth and stabilizing your blood sugar. They are naturally sweet, so if you freeze them they have the ability to make you feel like you're enjoying a frozen treat. When craving sugar, a handful of grapes can absolutely alleviate your desire. Take time to suck on and enjoy each frozen grape to further help kick that craving.

Making a plant-based smoothie, packed full of fruits, vegetables, and a healthy nut butter can not only help boost your intake of fresh foods daily but also curb sugar cravings. Having a smoothie can make you feel like you are having a delicious dessert shake, except without the unwanted sugar. The boost in fruit, veggie, and healthy fat intake also helps ensure adequate nutrition intake as well.

Another option is cinnamon, a sweet spice that can stop sugar cravings when nothing else can. It cures your sweet tooth by tricking your body into thinking you've had sugar! Cinnamon has been proven in research to help reduce sugar cravings by controlling blood glucose levels. This minimizes insulin spikes after meals that lead to more hunger and consuming even more sugar. Add some in your tea, coffee, or oatmeal, or take it in supplement form for an extra boost![20]

Fermented foods and drinks increase the body's immune system and can help regulate appetite and reduce sugar cravings. Foods such as tempeh, pickles, yogurt, and kimchi can all help you refrain from sugar. Healthy fermented beverages such as kombucha (a fermented tea) can curb your sugar cravings by bringing the body back into balance so that it can heal itself, rather than focusing on one particular ailment. Kombucha is a powerful adaptogen, meaning it's a natural substance considered to help the body adapt to stress and to exert a normalizing effect upon bodily processes. (More about adaptogens later!) Find my most recent and highest quality fermented supplement recommendations at www.theorganiclifeblog.com/fermented-supplements.

Atomic Healing

To truly understand the enormous power that food has on our physical health and energy, we need to explore its impact on our cells. Carbohydrates, fats, and proteins are broken down inside your cells into components that enter the cellular powerhouses known as mitochondria. Mitochondria are responsible for converting energy from the food you ingest into usable "currency." Throughout this cellular journey, these macronutrients undergo a complex series of transformations, eventually combining with oxygen to generate adenosine triphosphate (ATP), the molecular energy currency behind all biological functions.

To give you an idea of ATP's life-sustaining importance, your body converts a volume of ATP equal to your entire weight *every single day.* The most important function of mitochondria is to produce energy. This energy-intensive process throws off an immense number of electrons within the mitochondria, resulting in constant exposure to free radicals—and rendering the mitochondria especially vulnerable to damage.

In 2007 a group of researchers reported a major (but little-known) breakthrough in our understanding of how mitochondrial dysfunction unfolds, and they explained what can be done to protect yourself against its lethal impact. They discovered that potentially deadly defects in human mitochondria, such as molecular decay and membrane injury, begin to appear (and can be observed!) nearly a decade before the onset of permanent damage to the DNA.[21]

Most important, their analysis implied that mitochondrial dysfunction is reversible, enabling the life and health of cells to be prolonged at an atomic level. The key lies in early intervention. Early intervention ensures optimal mitochondrial function before irreversible DNA damage occurs. Atomic healing starts at the cellular level. When we change our most basic cells, we change our whole structure—our entire bodies. This easily leads to changing our entire lives! We'll review the latest research so that we can form a set of tools that specifically target and enhance our atomic health and function.

Tune Up Your Health

Our mitochondria essentially determine the fate of our health. They respond to and remember every single thing we do, piece of food we ingest, cigarette we smoke, or bottle of beer we drink. They don't second guess. They respond to exercise—or laziness. They react to inner peace or rage. They play an important role in cell death and regeneration, essentially determining if (and when) we get cancer or chronic illness. They are the powerhouse of our genome.

One of the universal characteristics of cancer cells is that they have serious mitochondrial dysfunction. Cancer cells display radically decreased numbers of functional mitochondria. In fact, mitochondria can still function in cancer cells, but one of the operations that occur particularly in cancer cells is that they instantly become dependent on glucose (sugar). They're *not using* their mitochondria—even though they have mitochondria there! These cells make a radical metabolic switch. This is like if you went from being an organic raw vegan for twenty years to exclusively eating McDonald's Big Macs, overnight.

Dr. Otto Warburg, a physician with a PhD in chemistry, is recognized by most experts as the greatest biochemist of the twentieth century. He received a Nobel Prize in 1931 for his research on the metabolism of tumors in the body, including the relationship of sugar and carbs as a source of energy production in cancer cells versus other cells. High glucose levels have been shown to accelerate cancer cell growth in the end stages of some forms of cancer, and consumption of large amounts of sugar is thought to increase risk of certain kinds of cancer.

Muscles use glucose for energy, and our brain is the most important muscle of them all. If you've ever tried to make a difficult decision, maintain your concentration, or say no to a treat when you have low blood sugar, you know that the struggle is real.

When our mitochondria are unhealthy, they don't produce as much ATP as our cells need to be robust and to make our whole bodies healthy. Our energy levels are critically dependent on having vigorous mitochondria.

Here's where it gets interesting: As people deplete their willpower, it seems they also begin depleting their glucose levels (blood sugar). Studies have found that people had lower glucose levels after exerting their willpower than those who did not.[22] Since the brain is a powerful organ and needs energy to run, researchers proposed that hardworking brain cells may be using up glucose faster than it can be replenished when exercising self-control.[23]

Control your stress and you can control your mental willpower. This control will boost your mitochondria and protect your body from using up your glucose resources, not only protecting your health for the long term, but also curbing sugar cravings immediately. We can prevent long-term dis-ease and acquire healthier habits—all at once. The primary source of our health should be approaching life in a way that protects our mitochondria. No matter your age, sex, race, or health condition, it's never too late to start. If you're human, read on. There are simple ways to tune up your health!

Safeguarding Our Cells with CoQ10

Coenzyme Q10 (CoQ10) safeguards mitochondria from age-related decay and cell death in a major way. First, CoQ10 is essential in the electron transport chain, aiding in the transfer of ATP so that it can be used in your cells. Ninety-five percent of all cellular energy relies on the amount of CoQ10 that your mitochondria have available to use.

Ubiquinol is an active form of CoQ10 that is naturally produced in our bodies and has been shown to have quite powerful antioxidant potential. Optimal mitochondrial function relies on a variety of cofactors, including CoQ10 functions. CoQ10 is particularly interesting because it not only supports the mitochondrial respiratory chain but also acts as a powerful antioxidant in mitochondrial membranes. CoQ10 is also found congregating in the same organs that have the highest mitochondrial density, such as the liver, kidneys, and heart.

Pharmaceutical medications have been heavily reported to affect liver, kidney, and heart function. These three organs are where oxidative stress and mitochondrial function are most important. The heart contains the highest concentration of mitochondria in the body, and it has the highest mitochondrial density. In essence, these organs need the most love.

Oral supplementation of coenzyme Q10 (or ubiquinol, which can be more easily absorbed for people over the age of forty and stays in the blood eight times longer) increases plasma production, lipoprotein, and blood vessel levels. This improves blood flow, heart rate, and organ function. It is claimed that Coenzyme Q10 supplementation also has the ability to play positive roles in treating some conditions of cardiovascular disease, neurodegenerative diseases, cancer, and diabetes. It can be a great help for skin problems, muscular dystrophy, proper brain function, cardiovascular function, blood flow, and life extension. It's also been shown to promote a speedy recovery from over-exercising.[24]

You'll be particularly susceptible to CoQ10 deficiency if you're taking statins for heart issues or as a preventive for heart conditions. Studies have shown that the use of cholesterol-lowering medications known as HMG-CoA reductase inhibitors (statins) decrease your circulating levels of coenzyme Q10. Therefore coenzyme Q10 supplementation might provide a great health benefit to some patients taking these sort of drugs—or patients looking to replace these drugs with a safe alternative. Be sure to research your alternative medications to determine that they are from a safe and reputable source.

CoQ10 is important for fighting free radicals, as tissue levels of coenzyme Q10 have been reported to decline with age. One of the hallmarks of aging is a decline in energy metabolism in many tissues, especially liver, heart, and skeletal muscle. It has been proposed that age-associated declines such as a pain, discomfort, signs of aging, and loss of elasticity may play a role in this decline and be related to CoQ10 deficiency. So if you want to look and feel younger, start taking this supplement! Organic supplements can be easily found online or at your local health food store, or your local grocery store or pharmacy. You only need to take one tablet a day to see results. Also try purchasing organic beauty products that contain CoQ10 as an ingredient for skin boosting rejuvenation.

ADAPTOGENS FOR PREVENTION

Adaptogens promote homeostasis in the body, decreasing cellular activity to stress while increasing energy. They have been shown to treat a wide variety of medical conditions, from chronic fatigue to cancer. They also increase your resistance to bacteria and infection and have a stabilizing effect on the body.

The metastatic process that encourages cancer growth can be categorized into three stages:

1. Tumor cell invasion into the surrounding tissue

2. Entering into blood or lymphatic vessels

3. Exiting into a new host environment (cancer spreading)

In many cases, metastatic cells undergo what's termed an epithelial–mesenchymal transition (EMT), where genetic and epigenetic (environmental genetic) events cause a polarized cell to become aggressive and invasive. In this state, cancer forms. Breast cancer is the most common cancer among women in the United States and the most common form of cancer in women of all races. The vast majority of breast cancer patient deaths are attributed to metastatic disease, where the primary tumor has invaded other sites in the body. Since these metastatic cells are often highly aggressive, difficult to detect, and chemo-resistant, a plant-based therapeutic strategy could be used to *prevent* metastatic disease as well as to treat it once it occurs.[25]

Withania somnifera (ashwagandha root powder) is one of the most popular Ayurvedic herbs composed of fourteen compounds known as withanolides, with withaferin A being the most prominent. Withaferin A inhibits tumor growth by targeting signaling proteins. Withaferin A treatment leads to cell cycle arrest and decreases reactive oxidative species (ROS). Excessive ROS production has been implicated in DNA mutations, aging, and cell death. Mitochondria-generated ROS play an important role in the release of proteins that your body needs to thrive. You can find ashwagandha at your local health food store or search for an organic supplement online. Buy it pure in bulk and add it in your teas, water, or food. Simply sprinkle on as a spice or garnish, or add hot water and cacao to your ashwagandha powder to make a healing tea.

Since the largely Indian manufacturers of Ayurvedic herbs are not regulated by the US Food and Drug Administration (FDA), be sure to research the source of any supplements you purchase. Before taking any new herbs or supplements, it's advisable to understand the real effects to make sure they're a good choice for you.

In a 2013 study conducted by Emory University ashwagandha extract was shown to be an incredible alternative to conventional medicine when used to prevent cancer growth. In their study, ashwagandha extract reduced tumor incidence and volume in breast cancer in mice and enhanced their life span. In humans, studies indicated it inhibited motility of breast cancer cells and thus inhibited cancer cell metastasis in patients who already had cancer.[26]

Ashwagandha is one of the most powerful adaptogens in the plant world. It's been called Indian ginseng for its uncanny ability to stimulate as well as regulate. In addition to being a powerful cancer fighter, it reduces blood sugar levels, boosts brain function, and helps our bodies and brains to fight symptoms of anxiety and depression. Studies have also revealed that ashwagandha may help reduce cortisol levels. Healthy cortisol levels enable the body to deal with stress and build the immune system. In a controlled study of chronically stressed adults, the group that supplemented with ashwagandha had significantly greater reductions in cortisol than the control group. The group taking the highest dose had a 30 percent reduction, on average.[27]

Another study conducted in 2012 found that those who received 1,250 mgs of ashwagandha had a total body improvement, including a total body fat reduction. Their lipids (fats) lowered, their quality of sleep improved, and without any added exercise, their muscles strengthened as well.[28] The traditional use of ashwagandha as an antianxiety, antitumor, anti-inflammatory, and antidepressant alternative has a solid scientific base.

What If I'm Pregnant?

While CoQ10 and ashwagandha have amazing health benefits, be sure to consult your doctor if you are pregnant or planning to become pregnant. There has not been sufficient research on the safety of CoQ10 supplementation during pregnancy, and your natural levels of coenzyme Q10 often increase during pregnancy. Ashwagandha should also be avoided during pregnancy because it may cause miscarriage at the wrong dosage. If you are taking either of these supplements or wish to take them and are pregnant, make sure you are monitored by a professional.

Exercise Your Way to Wellness

In addition to mindful nutrition and WILD food habits, getting enough exercise every day is crucial to your overall physical health and well-being. Physical *in*activity is the primary cause of most chronic diseases. Where there is stagnation, there is lifelessness. We benefit more from movement than we often expect. When you make changes on the outside, you'll always see those changes reflected on the inside, too. Change your sedentary habits and you can easily improve and prolong your life. You can be looking at a long, prosperous, and healthy future—if you keep active. The largest physical changes come with your movement. It's difficult to change your diet, form new habits, or be inspired to change your life if you don't move.

In 2012 a doctor from the University of Missouri, Columbia, a doctor from the University of California, Los Angeles, and a doctor from the Centre for Inflammation and Metabolism in Copenhagen came together in order to find out the major cause of chronic disease.[29] They noted that chronic diseases are major killers in the modern era. The question they asked was *why? What was the primary cause?*

They examined health in three stages:

1. They gathered historical health data to find out the existing evidence of links between chronic disease and personal habits throughout recorded time.

2. They sought to probe preventive medicine. That is, they scoured studies on preventive medicine to find out which modes of prevention in chronic disease had been shown to work time and time again, without fail. They studied prevention in chronic illness and disease including sarcopenia, metabolic syndrome, obesity, insulin resistance, prediabetes, type 2 diabetes, nonalcoholic fatty liver disease, coronary heart disease, peripheral artery disease, hypertension, stroke, congestive heart failure, endothelial dysfunction, arterial dyslipidemia, hemostasis, deep vein thrombosis, cognitive dysfunction, depression and anxiety, osteoporosis, osteoarthritis, balance, bone fracture/falls, rheumatoid arthritis, colon cancer, breast cancer, endometrial cancer, gestational diabetes, pre-eclampsia, polycystic ovary syndrome, erectile dysfunction, pain, diverticulitis, constipation, and gallbladder diseases. That covers a lot, in case you're counting.

3. The article concluded with the careful consideration of risk factors in longer-term sedentary groups, such as the clinical consequences of an inactive childhood/adolescence or state laws and public policy that might make it difficult for someone to exercise (those living in cities versus rural areas).

What they discovered is that the body rapidly becomes maladapted due to insufficient physical activity. If lack of movement is continued, there is a conclusive and substantial decrease in both total and quality years of life. Taken together, all departments of evidence show that physical inactivity is one important cause of most chronic diseases. In addition, physical activity primarily prevents or delays chronic diseases, implying that chronic disease does not need to be an inevitable outcome during life.

Daily movement has even been proven to prevent injury later on in life! A study conducted in 2017 by the University of California Irvine and Kaiser Permanente recently illustrated that those who exercised in their sixties and seventies were 35 to 45 percent less likely to have injuries from falling when they reached their nineties.[30] Remarkably, those with fewer injuries reported exercising just thirty minutes per day *a quarter century earlier!*

Lifestyle modification is extremely relevant for people who suffer from mental illness, and yet it's an often neglected intervention when we talk about mental health care. Running, cycling, yoga, jogging, swimming, and even mild exercise like walking, light yoga, breathing exercises, gardening, and dancing have been proven to reduce anxiety and depression. The physiological influence is significant: The communication between the body and the mind improves, moods are boosted, and endorphins are released. A bout of exercise not only releases our happy chemicals but also allows our minds to clear so that we can better handle stress and anxiety. If we do this every day, we're giving ourselves a brand-new chance every twenty-four hours to better deal with our lives. Health benefits of regular exercise include better sleep, improvement in mood, stress reduction, increased interest in sex, more endurance, less tiredness, and weight reduction. Decreased cholesterol and improved cardio fitness are also noticeable bonuses.

In 2004, researchers Lynette Craft and Frank Perna conducted a study on how exercise affects clinical depression.[31] Databases the researchers searched were Medline, PsycLit, PubMed, and SPORT-Discus from the time span of 1996 to 2003, using the terms *clinical depression, depression, exercise,* and *physical activity.* They noted that involvement in structured exercise has undoubtedly shown promise in alleviating symptoms of clinical depression in study after study. One study noted that just thirty minutes of treadmill walking for ten consecutive days was sufficient to produce a clinically relevant and statistically significant reduction in depression (a reduction of 6.5 points from baseline on the Hamilton Rating Scale for Depression, a multiple item questionnaire used to measure depression as well as recovery).[32] Research also suggests that the benefits of exercise involvement may be long lasting. In another study considered in the research by Craft and Perna, depressed adults who took part in a fitness program displayed significantly greater improvements in depression, anxiety, and self-concept than those in a control group after 12 weeks of training. The exercise participants also maintained many of these gains through the 12-month follow-up period.

The trick is to move every day, even if you feel like you can't. There is a marked difference between what we think we can do versus what we can actually do! Often, we find we're capable of a lot more than we think.

Twenty minutes of concentrated movement per day is all you need. More is better, but twenty minutes is a great starting point. Find the time to move—seriously. Traditional exercise—walking, hiking, short jogs, weight training, or yoga—is one of the most incredible things you can do for your health. No matter how much mind-work you're doing, it will never have a significant positive effect on your health if you aren't spending some time connecting with your body.

Inspired by my own at-home journey into fitness, I have designed fitness plans specifically for people to be able to exercise easily at home (you can find them at www.theorganiclifeblog.com/

fitness). The 14 Day Fitness Plan is made to transform your body in two weeks! Getting just twenty minutes of cardiovascular exercise a day (you can do it during one of your favorite Netflix shows) has been proven to help hundreds of health issues, as well as aid you in expanding your lifespan!

⁓⁓⁓⁓

Changing your harmful health habits into healthy food and exercise habits is easier than you think when you incorporate the WILD Method. It is truly astonishing what a healing effect food can have on our bodies, especially our cells. Foods can have a powerful impact not only on our physical health but also on our emotional and mental health. And a mere twenty minutes of exercise each day can dramatically improve your health and prevent chronic disease. Remember, good nutrition plus exercise plus meditation can lead to a better life. Trust your intuition and use mind-strengthening techniques like meditation to help you stay the course.

CHAPTER 9

The Medicine Cabinet:
Natural Alternatives to Painkillers

I can honestly say that pharmaceutical drugs were my longest and most toxic relationship—hands down. I realized that I had blindly accepted the idea that I needed pharmaceutical drugs for most of my life. I had never before questioned the idea that they were the answer. Then I faced an uncomfortable reality: the idea of needing drugs for my feelings, pain, and problems was outdated. It hadn't worked for me in the near dozen years since I'd first tried it. My body hated drugs.

It's still hard for me to rattle off the names of everything I had been prescribed without forgetting one or two. At the time I was taking them, it was difficult for me to recall what many of the drugs were even for or how long I had been on them. I figured that my doctors had done their due diligence and that none of these drugs were interacting with one another and harming me.

I was dead wrong.

Even more frightening, I was nowhere close to grasping the idea that many of the pharmaceutical drugs I took were *possibly deadly* when combined.

There is nothing cool, sexy, trendy, or heroic about the withdrawal that followed my decision to quit my meds cold turkey. It totally fucking sucked. Pharmaceutical withdrawal is no joke, and you do not need to be on drugs for eleven years to experience it. Although you may only take your drugs on a short-term basis, you may experience the same withdrawals that I did, perhaps just not for as long a period of time (or perhaps for longer). I tried to work with doctors to withdraw, but any doctor that I saw told me that what I was doing (coming off my drugs) was "a symptom of my illness," and they each tried to put me on more or different drugs. This is common.

It was a horrible idea for me, especially after a decade-plus-long drug habit. My body wasn't just craving the drugs, my body needed the drugs. It wasn't your average detox. I went through more than three years of withdrawals that were worse than opiate, alcohol, and meth withdrawals combined. (I wrote about this extensively in my first book, *Cured by Nature*, if you're inclined to learn more about exactly what withdrawal entails.)

If you choose to wean yourself off of medications, read on to find methods that will help you to taper off slowly with help from your family, friends, and medical professionals. While I did this on my own, cold turkey, I DO NOT RECOMMEND THIS. You must be extremely careful when you decide to stop taking prescription medication, and it's best to do it gradually while being monitored by a professional. Find a doctor who will work *with* you and *for* you. If you choose detox as a method of treatment, find a naturopath and a different doctor in the same field who will work with you to taper off your drugs slowly. It is extremely dangerous to come off your drugs suddenly—and it can kill you. Never (ever, ever, ever) taper off or come off your drugs without consulting a doctor.

If your doctor dissuades you, find a support system (you have a whole tribe over at The Organic Life—we have resources like a private Facebook group and a running list of naturopaths and professionals in holistic fields). Find another doctor. Do your research and don't give up. There are a lot more resources out there now than there were just seven years ago when I first started my journey. Books I can recommend besides my own that deal with this concept include *How to Heal Yourself When No One Else Can* by Amy Scher, *You Can Heal Your Life* by Louise Hay, *Quantum Healing* by Deepak Chopra, and *Prescription for Nutritional Healing* by Phyllis A. Balch.

In this chapter I will provide some helpful guidelines for those who wish to decrease their prescription drug use. I will also explain some of the dangers of pain medications that you may not even know about, as well as their ramifications for your physical health. So often a pill is the first line of defense when we encounter a problem—we see it as a quick and easy solution to many types of pain. Unfortunately, as you'll see, this quick fix is an illusion. It's a short-term solution to a permanent problem. Eventually it wears off, or perhaps never works at all, leaving us in even more pain unless we increase our dosage or find an alternative solution. But if you are in physical pain, there is hope. There are so many natural alternatives that provide real and lasting relief.

Pain Prescriptions Prevent Healing

Picture this: You head to the doctor and tell her you have persistent back pain. She listens and then prescribes you the most common treatment available today, a medication meant to treat your pain. You take the medication starting that day, and for a little while you are happy to be experiencing some relief. However, weeks later you notice that your pain is actually increasing. . . . *How could this be?*

Most anti-inflammatory medications today are categorized as Nonsteroidal Anti-Inflammatory Drugs (NSAIDS) or Cox-2 inhibitors, and they're not actually treating your pain—they're *blocking* it. When your back now tries to send the signal I AM IN PAIN to your brain, these drugs stop that message in its tracks. In other words, your pain could be increasing, and you would be oblivious to it. Worse, this one-size-fits-all method of treatment *doesn't* promote healing—it prevents it.

Over time, Cox-2 inhibitors have been proven to *increase* pain, increase risk of heart attack, and they may cause allergic reactions (in patients who never had allergies before!). Common NSAID drugs, like Celebrex and Vioxx, may increase the risk of serious, sometimes even fatal, stomach and intestinal reactions such as bleeding, ulcers, and perforation of the stomach or intestines.

This is legal? Surprisingly, yes. Initially, the United States Food and Drug Administration (FDA) asked Vioxx to add a warning label to their product. They did, but eventually the FDA took Vioxx off the market altogether because resulting lawsuits alleged heart attacks, strokes, and even death from the drug. Many suspect that the Merck pharmaceutical company and the FDA worked together to keep the drug on the market and quiet many thousands of health concerns over the years. By that point, more than 38,000 deaths were related to Vioxx use and up to 25 million Americans had taken the drug. I should know. I was one of the 25 million people who took Vioxx until it was taken off the market, and then I was one of the people immediately prescribed Celebrex (another drug manufactured by Merck) as an alternative drug option to treat my back pain. In 2011 Merck plead guilty and paid a massive $950 million settlement to the US government and 43 states over the way it deceptively marketed Vioxx as a painkiller.[33] Ironically, they barely took a hit. Merck made an annual revenue of over $48 billion that year.

Almost everyone who takes a pill for their ailments does so for the same reason: They believe it will help them. But many folks don't know *why* they're taking what they're taking. Many good people who want to get better don't recognize that the pharmaceutical industry is a business and they have a target customer: You.

Some drugs are necessary, of course. Even psychiatric drugs, in severe cases. But look at the numbers, and there's just no doubt that we're overmedicated. On record, Walgreens sold over 900 million—almost a billion—prescription drugs in 2015. That's three times more drugs than there are people in this country! Walgreens sold enough drugs that year for everyone in the US—man, woman, and child—to be on three separate medications at the same time. What makes this number so jaw-dropping? *That's just one pharmacy!!* These companies have investors, stockholders, lobbyists, and CFOs to satisfy. Their filled prescription drug numbers WILL go up, year by year. I have no doubt about that, and their books and company strategies prove it.

We need to know what we can do for ourselves to make sure we're not one of the overmedicated ones. Unfortunately, we have a long history of seeing pills as medicine and believing that they will cure our ailments.

The History of "Medicine"

Today, when most people hear the word "medicine," they most likely think of a diagnosis, a drug, or a treatment. But, in fact, medicine has a colorful history that begins as early as prehistoric man. The word medicine is derived from Latin *medicus*, meaning "physician." The study encompasses a variety of practices and treatments in our culture, such as biomedical sciences, genetics, drugs, and radiation. Its meaning has changed many times. The use of medicine dates to the evolution of our species, where evidence of plant-based healing, blood-letting, and trepanning (skull drilling) has been uncovered. The history of medicine is pockmarked with debunked theories, painful medieval practices (did I mention skull drilling?), and unexplainable recoveries and reversals. It's far more complicated than most of us realize, and this is why it's important to do your research.

Speaking of skull drilling, the 1920s version of you would have likely received a proper lobotomy for all those pesky anxious and stressful feelings we all admittedly suffer from today. Lobotomies were the most popular medical practice of the time! A lobotomy, in case you aren't up on your hip vintage medical terms, is a medical procedure that involves damaging frontal brain tissue in order to treat mental illness or anxiety. It requires a doctor to drill through both of the eye sockets of his patient with two ten-inch picks and damage his or her (her, most of the time) frontal neurons. The idea was that if you damaged that part of the brain, you could stop bad behavior. The inventor of the ever-popular lobotomy was given a Nobel Prize in 1949. Enough said.

In the past, various forms of medicine have been considered everything from an art form and a science to witchcraft and complete quackery. Beauty treatments like the ever-popular clay mask, as well as bizarre medical practices like lobotomies were commonplace to the ancient Egyptians. Their top medical treatments included using crocodile dung for contraception and placing dead mice on their teeth to ward off toothache. Gross!

Babies in the 1920s were soothed with cough syrups that contained morphine, cannabis indica, heroin, and chloroform. Heroin was originally developed by Bayer, the same people who developed aspirin in the 1890s and make your favorite "fast-acting" Tylenol. Bayer and two other German pharmaceutical and chemical companies also formed the giant conglomerate company called IG Farben that funded Hitler's elections and his reign, and the company became the largest single profiteer of the Second World War.

At the 1947 IG Farben Trial, one of the Nuremberg proceedings held by the United States to prosecute major German war criminals, thirteen directors of IG Farben were sentenced to jail terms for their war crimes, and twenty-four were arraigned. But all defendants who were sentenced received early release. Some went on to be heads of major companies, and the Bayer company survived the Allies' liquidation of IG Farben.

While medicine's history is also pockmarked with debunked theories and bizarre practices, it's important to note that many of the most common ailments we face today—pain, anxiety, inflammation, insomnia, acne, and more—have all been successfully treated for thousands of years. Before the modern pharmaceutical industry came along, medicine doctors, scientists, shamans, healers, and philosophers ruled. They discovered one thing in common: The answers to our most common problems are all around us. Your real medicine is in the earth you stand on. Real medicine is the food we eat.

Did you ever stop to think that even though you pick them up at the drug store, somewhere along the line you are placated into thinking about pharmaceutical drugs as medicine—and not as drugs? By very definition, you can create your own medicine. *You* are meant to be the *medicus*—the physician. There is real help out there—if you know where to look for it. When you start deciding what supports your body and what does not, you can begin the most effective process of healing through your very own choices.

Healing Your Gut

Your medicine cabinet may be a shelf in your bathroom decorated with a smattering of orange bottles. Or it might be your fridge full of healing foods or your pantry stocked with supplements. Your form of medicine might be a decision you make to wake up earlier, take a run, or make a healthy, vibrant meal.

Your gut creates ten times more serotonin than your brain. Many doctors believe that at times flooding the gut with SSRIs (serotonin reuptake inhibitors, most commonly prescribed for depression, which dissolve in the stomach) can actually *negatively* impact your body's ability to deal with stress or depression because they disrupt the sophisticated neural network responsible for transferring clear messages to your body and brain.

There is strong evidence that most of your health begins in your gut. In just the last few years, evidence has mounted from studies in rodents that their gut microbes can influence neural development, brain chemistry, and a wide range of behavioral phenomena, including (but not limited to) emotional behavior, pain perception, and how the stress system responds. And that's just rats![34]

This implies that if we heal the gut (and we'll talk about how in this book!), we can heal the mind. Ask yourself: How can blocking your pain, masking anxieties, labeling quirks, and putting a Band-Aid on your moods *really* be helping you?

TIPS FOR TAKING PRESCRIPTION DRUGS

Here are some personal tips if you are choosing or considering pharmaceutical medication as a treatment:

- As a first step in taking control of your health, always ask your doctor to explain your ailment until you understand it. Then inquire about *how* (exactly) the pills they've prescribed for you are helping your body to treat whatever your ailment is.

- Ask your doctor if he or she knows of any natural alternatives that do the same thing as the pills they are prescribing you. Ask what your medication's "natural alternative" is—that is, what plant the medication is inspired by. For instance, Valium's natural derivative is valerian. Aspirin's (acetylsalicylate) natural alternative is willow bark (*Salix*). Sometimes they even sound similar in their clinical names.

- Along the way, I would encourage you to question *why* you are choosing the route you are for your personal healing, and if it's truly helping you in the way that you expected. Every day, ask yourself at least once: *Have I explored every possible route for recovery? Am I improving? Is this my peak self?*

- Before you ever fill another prescription, write down a list of what you expect from that medication. Then, compare that list with how you *truly feel* over the course of your treatment. This way you can see if the drugs are actually meeting your expectations, or if your expectations change based on how the drugs are working.

- Always do your own research about any drug a doctor prescribes you before you ever fill another prescription again. It's your right. This research is best done at the library.

- Search for forums of people who have used the drug (and come off the drug!) and experienced real effects.

- Question everything. It's the only way to figure out your personal path to healing.

The Real Remedies

Change feeds our growth. Without change, we can't learn and we can't get better. Growth is what propels us forward and gives us purpose. The only lesson we learn when getting a label and a prescription is to take a pill for our problems.

Anxious? Take a pill.

In pain? Take a pill.

Uncomfortable? Take a pill.

This is damaging to us in two major ways. First, it's not giving us the opportunity for change and growth that we truly need to have a purposeful, peaceful life. When we take a pill for our feelings and don't do the inner work, we mask the problem instead of addressing it. We confuse our body instead of healing our body. Rather than restoring us, this depletes us. Second, by taking a pill when we're in pain or uncomfortable, we're confirming and constantly reinforcing to our body that this is the correct way to deal with our problems. Instead of overcoming our challenges and growing mentally, we're actually suppressing these challenges that our brains and our bodies *need* to advance and adapt. The new person we are—or could become—gets drowned out. These are the only kind of challenges that truly help us to grow.

Learning from our experiences and making decisions to claim our power is so essential to our growth as people and our growth as a human race. When we give away all our power to medication alone, all the new neural pathways we need to form to cope with our problems become stifled. All the inspiration we need to find our healthiest self gets completely drowned out by what pharmaceuticals are doing to our delicate neurons. Life gets cloudier, instead of clearer, and every new drug is another Band-Aid on top of another broken bone.

Drugs are necessary, of course, but they are not the only answer. Some of the time they can help in miraculous ways. Antibiotics, for instance, have saved many lives. But in too many cases antibiotics are overprescribed or prescribed when they are not needed. For instance, many dermatologists recommend Minocycline (an antibiotic) for the treatment of hormonal acne. Side effects include dizziness, vertigo (which is particularly common), and headaches due to increased cranial pressure. That's right: Minocycline can swell your brain, and by the way, it only works on mild to moderate acne.

Hormonal acne is triggered by (you guessed it!) hormones—not "clogged pores" or bacterial buildup (which Minocycline claims to attack). On top of Minocycline not addressing your hormones, your body easily builds up tolerances to antibacterial drugs, so flooding your system with these drugs unnecessarily creates more complications for your health and wellness down the road. Too often medications create many more issues for us than they solve. Doctors frequently prescribe medication to their patients who don't need it at all!

If you're going to take something for your discomfort, pain, or anxiety anyway, why not take something that supports your body, instead of weakening it? We can catch our harmful habits and harness them to start working for us—instead of working against us.

What if I told you that the solution to your acne, your skin problems, and your hormone balance lay in a single safe supplement? A supplement derived from plants that not only clears your skin but also balances your hormones and actually supports your health, including warding off certain cancers? Those with hormonal acne or hormonal imbalances associated with menstruation, PMS, perimenopause, menopause, or postmenopause may benefit immensely from this supplement, as it balances hormones, supports "good estrogen," gets rid of "bad estrogen," and can even be a substitute for HRT (hormone replacement therapy)!

This is not blind optimism or fiction. This supplement exists. It's called DIM (we'll cover this miraculous herb in chapter 11!) and has saved many complexions, including my own.

Regardless of if we're choosing medication for treatment, we should be incorporating natural methods of healing into our everyday lives. The reason it's important to have natural methods and tools for healing is because at the end of the day, you can't rely on a pill. A pill won't do the work. You need to do the work, and you're the only one who can. You need to be able to rely on yourself, no matter what.

How would a surgeon perform an operation if there was a cast covering your leg? She couldn't. She would need to remove the cast first to see how bad the problem was before she could even begin to help you. Having the cast there may have provided some temporary relief for you mentally, but it does nothing to heal you.

Each one of us is born with the capacity to heal, to grow, and to change. That's how you got to where you are right now. You've continually adapted. We're here to live our best life, no matter what circumstances we're born into. Our ability to accomplish our dreams is not based on our past experience. Our success—in health, business, family, or our spiritual practice—is based on our willingness to embrace a new future. If you want real help, this is all you need to do.

There is a better way—and it has a proven past. Ancient healing remedies have worked for centuries. Long before there was "modern" or what we now consider "Western" medicine, people still got sick and still had to be treated. Ancient people had incredible healing secrets that worked for thousands of years before Big Pharma came along. Those same cures still work for us today!

Natural Alternatives to Pain Killers

If you're suffering from a toothache, backache, or any other type of pain, your first impulse might be to reach for a pill. Many people rely on medications to treat their discomfort every day, but they come with the risk of real effects such as loss of coordination, drowsiness, aggression, drug interactions, and the distinct possibility of becoming habit-forming.

Opiate addiction has reached record highs in the United States. It is estimated that as many as 36 million people abuse prescription painkillers worldwide,[35] and emergency room visits related to opiate use nearly tripled in just the four years from 2004 to 2008 in the United States.[36]

I used to slap fentanyl patches on my skin for my pain. Fentanyl is considered deadlier than heroin, because it takes less of it to kill you. Three milligrams of fentanyl is enough to kill an average-sized adult male. A lethal dose of heroin is about thirty milligrams—ten times that amount! The drug overdose death statistics in 2016 reached upwards of 65,000—the largest jump ever recorded in US history, according to the *New York Times,* in large part due to an influx of opioid drugs like fentanyl.[37] All evidence shows that problems have continued to worsen.

The state of Ohio recently filed a lawsuit against the pharmaceutical industry after publicly declaring pharmaceutical opioid death tolls a "national epidemic."[38] In the suit, they charged the drug companies with spending "millions of dollars on promotional activities and materials that falsely deny or trivialize the risks of opioids while overstating the benefits of using them for chronic pain." By 2012, the suit says, opioid prescriptions in Ohio equaled 68 pills a year for every resident of the state, including children. Defendants in the case include Purdue Pharma (which makes OxyContin), Teva Pharmaceutical Industries (who paid out $1.6 million to the state of California in 2017 after losing a similar suit), Johnson & Johnson, Endo Pharmaceuticals, Allergan, and others.

We don't have to take this risk! Chronic pain affects about a third of the US population. Roughly 20 percent of America was prescribed an opioid in 2016.[39] But you don't have to be someone who risks their life to cure their pain! I am not a slave to addictive drugs any longer, despite still suffering from occasional arthritic inflammation. Today, I use natural alternatives to the deadly painkillers I once took.

I regularly create teas and meals with anti-inflammatory, anti-spasmodic spices. I hand-pour potions of coconut milk, skullcap herb, valerian root, and California poppy, which have all been proven for long-lasting pain relief. I watch my body respond by relaxing, unwinding, and then having the energy to move and not remain stagnant. I can feel my muscles strengthening as well as loosening. There are days I can feel pain creeping up, and now I have a way to combat it immediately. With just a few tweaks and my go-to natural remedies, I am pain-free in no time!

Below are your best natural alternatives to the most commonly prescribed painkillers. The best part is you probably already have many of them in your kitchen or backyard! Many of the foods can be incorporated into your life every day—or every day for as long as you experience pain or discomfort. You can enjoy the herbal teas as needed, for example during the week you experience PMS. All of the herbal supplements come with their own instructions depending

PAINKILLERS AND THEIR SIDE EFFECTS

Commonly Prescribed Painkiller Medication:

Oxycodone, Percocet, Lyrica, Norco, OxyContin, Dilaudid, Vicodin, Aleve, Naproxen, Codeine, Morphine, Celebrex, Vioxx, Demerol, Lortab, Palladone, Tramadol, Tylenol

Negative Side Effects from Painkiller Drugs:

Constipation, nausea, vomiting, dizziness, confusion, addiction, respiratory problems, unconsciousness, increased sensitivity to pain, physical dependence, dry mouth, rash, liver damage, itching, sweating, low testosterone, kidney damage, ulcers, miscarriage, coma, and death upon the brand, so you can follow the dosage recommendations listed on the bottles without any worry of "overdose." You can find more natural pain relief options and keep up with my new finds at www.theorganiclifeblog.com/pain-relief.

Ginger

Ginger has quite the history of pain relief. It has been commonly used since the dawn of Ayurveda and was described as "the beverage of the holiest spirits" by the ancient Koreans. Today, medical journals have found that a few tablespoons of ginger a day helps ease muscle pain.

Ginger works on a cellular level because it contains anti-inflammatory, anti-ulcer, and antioxidant agents as well as analgesic (inflammation-fighting) properties. Ginger has been shown to reduce cytokines (inflammation-causing substances that are often linked to pain) by breaking down existing inflammation in the joints—naturally!

Use ginger every day for chronic daily pain. You can buy raw ginger and put pieces into a tea strainer, boil hot water, and drink it as a tea. You can add fresh, raw ginger to a juice or smoothie and even incorporate it into your meals. Add it on top of noodles, salad, soup, or sushi. You can also buy premade ginger tea or supplemental ginger vitamins—there are also sugar-free ginger chews for those of us with a sweet tooth. They work equally well!

Turmeric

Used for more than four thousand years, turmeric boosts more than just your moods, as we touched on earlier in the Prozac vs. turmeric study. A member of the ginger family, it's an effective anti-inflammatory that can help with joint problems, circulation and arthritis. It's been used to treat rheumatoid and osteoarthritis pain straight at the source.

Turmeric is also one of the easiest herbs to incorporate into your daily routine: Add it to meals, smoothies, teas or take it as a capsule. Joints feel more fluid after use, and it can replace common NSAIDS used for pain and inflammation. Include turmeric in your meals every day when you are struggling with joint pain.

Chamomile

Chamomile extract is a powerful pain reliever that can soothe aches at the source by lubricating joints and inhibiting bone loss. It's also been shown to help ease menstrual cramps and has been globally promoted as a relaxation herb for thousands of years. It has anxiolytic properties, meaning that it naturally inhibits anxiety.

Plus, you can find chamomile practically everywhere: the grocery store, coffee shop or even your local diner will likely have options for chamomile tea. Speaking as someone who's sensitive to caffeine, I can attest that it's the most common caffeine-free tea available today. You can take chamomile as a tea, a tincture, or a supplement. Also look for chamomile in your skincare. It's the perfect ingredient for fighting skin inflammation and calming painful cysts from acne, rashes from eczema, and flare-ups from psoriasis. When used in skincare, chamomile leaves you with less inflamed skin and a golden glow, reminiscent of the sunny-colored flower itself.

Garlic

Egyptians worshipped it. Entire literary genres have been written about it. It was even used as currency in previous centuries!

While these may not be your very first thoughts about garlic, this powerful plant contains naturally occurring antioxidants that are amazing for fighting discomfort, arthritis, cancer, and heart disease. It's great for healthy joints and pain management. Simply toss a few cloves of garlic into your tea strainer, boil water, and drink with some honey. You can also add it to your fresh juice or blender for a smoothie, as well as many of your meals—it acts powerfully on the body if you cook with it. You can also put garlic cloves in your bath as aromatherapy. Garlic works wonders for long-term pain relief and there is no chance of an "overdose" on this powerful plant. (I mean, maybe your significant other might think so if you come in for the smooch one too many times without brushing, but trust me, your body will thank you!)

Devil's Claw

Devil's claw is incredible for pain management—it remains one of my personal staples. Devil's claw can be used to treat so many issues including arthritis, gout, muscle pain, back pain, tendonitis, chest pain, gastrointestinal upset or heartburn, fever, and migraine headaches. It is also used for difficulties in childbirth, menstrual problems, allergic reactions, loss of appetite, PMS, PMDD, and kidney and bladder disease. You can take it as a capsule, a tincture, a tea, or apply it directly to the pain site. Devil's claw has been proven to work just as well as NSAIDs.

In a randomized, double-blind, parallel group study conducted in France, patients received either capsules containing devil's claw or capsules containing a pharmaceutical NSAID drug.[40] Pain measurements of all patients indicated that those taking the herb and those patients taking the drug experienced similar benefits. However the study also revealed that patients taking devil's claw experienced

significantly *fewer* adverse real effects than those taking the pharmaceutical NSAID drug.

California Poppy

California poppy is an amazing natural painkiller that promotes
relaxation and acts as a nerve relaxer, sedative, analgesic, antispasmodic, anxiolytic, and antihistamine. Its antispasmodic properties relax muscles throughout the body, making it a useful remedy
for soothing tense, aching muscles and treating stress-related gut
problems, IBS, colic, and gallbladder pain. It slows a rapid heartbeat,
relieves palpitations, and reduces blood pressure. California poppy
has mind-enhancing properties and can also be useful in the treatment of behavioral disorders, such as ADD and ADHD, in children
and young adults.

This beautiful flower can be safely taken as a supplement, tincture, or tea for pain relief. Simply add the poppy seeds to a tea bag,
put the teabag into a teacup, add some honey, coconut milk, and
hot water, and enjoy!

Skullcap

The skullcap plant is one of the most useful herbs for pain ever to
be discovered. Skullcap relieves nervous tension and, unlike pharmaceuticals, actually restores optimal function to organs and tissues throughout the body. It is a powerful spasmolytic, meaning it
relieves and decreases muscle spasms.

Skullcap is specifically useful when someone has nervous,
emotional irritability. Nervous irritability sometimes shows up in
the body as skeletal muscle tension (neck and back), teeth grind-
ing, spasms, tremors, stress headaches, migraines, restlessness, and
agitation. Skullcap works naturally to soothe all of this tension. You
can take it in pill, tincture, or tea form.

Willow Bark

Common over-the-counter pain relievers have been prescribed to children and teens to treat mild pain for more than a hundred years. Most of these have been considered safe for this time, but aspirin is a glaring exception. Use of aspirin in children is specifically associated with the risk of Reye's syndrome. The symptoms of Reye's syndrome come on quickly and start with severe vomiting. Often children are given aspirin in the case of headaches or flus, so the first symptom may or may not raise alarms. This first red flag is followed by more dangerous symptoms, where children become confused and lethargic. Untreated, this can quickly lead to liver and brain swelling. Within hours, they may have seizures or fall into a coma.

If parents don't recognize the symptoms as Reye's syndrome, children can often lose their lives. What begins as a parent doing their best to try to help a child can turn into a nightmare scenario for even the most astute and educated of caretakers.

Folks have been using willow bark to ease inflammation (the cause of most aches and pains) for centuries. The chemical salicin, which is similar to the main ingredient in aspirin, is found in the bark of the white willow, and it works much the same way as aspirin, without any nasty real effects.

Originally, people chewed the bark itself to relieve pain and fevers. Now willow bark is sold as a dried herb that can be brewed as a tea. It also comes as a capsule or liquid supplement. Willow bark is commonly used to treat headache, fever, the common flu, cramps, back pain, spinal disease, osteoarthritis, rheumatoid arthritis, migraines, and many more conditions. Willow bark is safe for children, teens, and even dogs!*

---

* Always consult with your vet before giving your pets supplements.

How One Woman Used Natural Remedies
to Heal Her Pain

During the winter last year, Tina awoke one morning with muscle aches and fatigue all over her body. It persisted for more than two weeks and she became frustrated having to deal with the debilitating pain. She saw her primary care physician, and he ultimately diagnosed her with a condition called fibromyalgia. It's a disease of the central nervous system that manifests itself in all over body pain and chronic fatigue. The only accepted Western treatment available for this condition is powerful narcotics, so Tina's doctor referred her to a pain management specialist. When she arrived home, she called and made an appointment with the specialist right away.

Several days later, Tina met with the pain specialist. She explained her diagnosis, he confirmed it through a pressure point test, and Tina was handed a prescription for OxyContin, a powerful narcotic often used to treat fibromyalgia. Tina filled her prescription and took her first dose that day.

Her narcotic medicine worked for a short while, but Tina soon found strange symptoms pop up if she didn't take her pills every day: feelings of nausea, shakes, and dizziness. She realized after a few days that these were the symptoms of withdrawal. Her body was becoming addicted to the drugs. Without using them daily, she experienced no relief from her pain.

Tina stopped her pharmacological method of treatment and searched for a natural alternative. She came across my first book plus a handful of others that put her on the right track. Tina began walking with her Pomeranian KoKo every morning and using a heating pad if she felt inflammation creeping in. She began taking skullcap, turmeric, and devil's claw every morning as a hot tea. She'd prepare a turmeric latte and then add skullcap and devil's claw tinctures. Two droppers full of tincture and Tina had a powerful pain relief potion right in her teacup!

After using this new, plant-based method of healing for a year, Tina suffers from far fewer flare-ups, and when they do creep in, she has a go-to arsenal to cure her pain that works, time and time again. Tina creates her herbal concoction multiple times a day, as it provides her with the extensive pain relief that she sought when taking OxyContin. She has become a passionate advocate for a plant-based lifestyle, especially in people dealing with pain and inflammation. Luckily, Tina caught her harmful habit before it had taken over her life. When Tina contacted me, she had successfully switched her OxyContin habit to beautiful new WILD habits: taking morning walks, preparing healing teas, and using herbs to cure her pain. We can all do this—and now you know how!

Prescription drugs cause very real effects in our bodies, and many times these painkillers harm us more than they heal us, blocking our pain instead of treating it, and causing us to need higher dosages to achieve relief from our pain. While certain drugs are of course necessary, we are clearly overmedicated. Instead of relying on a pill to cure your aches and pains, consider one of the many natural healing remedies available in foods, herbs, teas, and supplements. In the next chapter we'll explore some additional natural alternatives for treating mental disorders.

CHAPTER 10

Nature's Mental Health Remedies

When I came off my meds, my mission was not to never take them again. I thought the natural remedies might work a little, but I wasn't expecting them to work better than the prescription drugs. I was incredibly surprised to find that many natural solutions provided the long-term effective relief that I had always been searching for, without the scary real effects I had experienced from pharmaceutical medications.

Many people are given antidepressants and antianxiety meds to address symptoms without knowing the real cause of the imbalance. This begs the question: With all these natural options available to us, are we unnecessarily overmedicating with pharmaceuticals? A quick look at the numbers may speak for itself. Let's start by reminding ourselves that Walgreens sold enough pharmaceuticals to put every man, woman, and child in this country on three drugs at the same time . . . and that's just one pharmacy.

Drugs may seem like a solution and can undoubtedly save lives in certain instances, but our addiction to prescription treatment is most likely masking our problem—not treating it. So many amazing healthy and natural alternatives exist for our health. Pills do not treat the underlying cause of our pain, our anxiety, or our moods. Nature does.

Nature has a medicine cabinet full of remedies for you to treat any health problem you have. You just need to open it.

Nature's Antidepressants

More than one-third of doctor's visits end with the patient leaving the office with a prescription in their hand. This makes medication the most common form of treatment in the United States. Since this phenomenon began, it's become increasingly important for us to incorporate vitamins, herbs, or supplements so that we can support our systems. Drugs change the way our bodies work—even if they've been prescribed to us.

Antidepressants are drugs used for the treatment of major depressive disorders, OCD, anxiety disorders, addiction, and more. They are often the first line of treatment used for clinical depression. Conflicting studies have arisen as to the effectiveness of antidepressant drugs in comparison with placebos. Researchers Irving Kirsch and Thomas Moore have contested that the evidence for the pharmacological use of antidepressants is consistent with that of placebos, suggesting that *just taking the drug* is what is making the patients feel better—not the drugs themselves.[41] Kirsch and Moore concluded that antidepressants do not pose a significant clinical effect for the treatment of depression. Their study included *unpublished* studies on pharmaceutical drugs done by the FDA.

One in three women who visit a doctor are prescribed an antidepressant medication. One in ten take at least one antidepressant drug. Interestingly, studies reveal that up to 70 percent of those taking an antidepressant *do just as well taking a placebo or sugar pill.*

Nature, on the other hand, has been providing us with natural antidepressants for years.

Below are some of the best natural alternatives to prescription antidepressants. They include amino acids, antioxidants, vitamins, and herbs. Follow the guidelines on the bottles of whichever remedies you choose to take and consult a naturopath, an internet source like Drugs.com/drug-interactions, and/or your doctor if you intend to take more than two supplements at a time. This way you know if there are possible interactions, which is especially important if you are taking pharmaceutical medication. Many of these remedies provide almost immediate relief within minutes to hours, so my recommendation is to slowly increase your dosage a bit before moving on to something new, if for any reason you feel they didn't work as hoped the first time. Unlike medication, there is no risk of overdosing on a plant or a tea, as long as you don't consume a toxic amount or deliberately make yourself sick (as you can do with any food or beverage). You can always learn about more natural antidepression options and keep up with my new finds at www.theorganiclifeblog.com/nodepression.

ANTIDEPRESSANTS AND THEIR SIDE EFFECTS

Commonly Prescribed Antidepressants and Mood Stabilizers

Prozac, Zoloft, Paxil, Celexa, Lexapro, Oleptro, MAO inhibitors, Tricyclics, Anafranil, Depakote, Lithium, Lamictal, Abilify, Cymbalta, Seroquel, Wellbutrin, Zyprexa

Negative Effects of Prescription Antidepressants

Trouble sleeping, nausea, insomnia, decreased libido, weight gain, erectile dysfunction, dry mouth, decreased orgasm, blurred vision, agitation, irritability, increase in anxiety, constipation, dizziness, headaches, sleepiness, increased appetite, stomach upset, nausea, drop in blood pressure, vertigo, increased sweating, increase in urinary tract infections

Natural Antidepressant Alternatives

GABA

GABA (gamma-aminobutyric acid) is a neurotransmitter that we've touched on a few times throughout this book already. I mentioned that it gets depleted when you take pharmacological drugs. GABA supplements support your neurotransmitters and balance your brain chemistry. If you feel as though life is flavorless or you have a hard time concentrating through a depressive brain fog, GABA is your answer. It is a neurotransmitter involved in inhibition and stress relief. Low GABA levels have been linked to depression and anxiety.

In fact, studies have proven that many antianxiety and anti-depressant medications actually suppress your GABA, making it harder for your body to naturally do the work to boost or manage your mood.

GABA is an amino acid that calms the nervous system and works almost like a natural, super-mellow tranquilizer. It is sold as a capsule, pill, or powder. You can take it in your tea or take capsules every day to support your moods and help fight anxiety and depression.

CoQ10

There is now evidence that major depression is accompanied by an induction of inflammatory and oxidative stress pathways. Coenzyme Q10 (CoQ10) is a strong antioxidant that has anti-inflammatory effects. As we discussed in chapter 8, CoQ10 is also needed to make ATP, the major energy source needed for cell growth. It is needed for maintenance and to power several of the body's biological processes, including brain function and regulating your mood.

A Belgian study conducted in 2009 showed that low CoQ10 plays a role in depression and suggests that depressed patients may benefit from CoQ10 supplementation.[42]

CoQ10 also functions as an antioxidant, protecting the body from damaging molecules. CoQ10 can be obtained via food sources or as a nutritional supplement. The foods highest in CoQ10 include salmon, sardines, and beef liver.

B Vitamins

Prescription antidepressants like Prozac and other selective serotonin reuptake inhibitors (SSRIs) focus on one neurotransmitter in particular: serotonin. The drugs claim to flood your system with this neurotransmitter. But evidence suggests that this "flooding" of serotonin is actually disrupting our gut and harming our body's ability to make, distribute, or create serotonin normally. This results in an uphill battle against depressive feelings. A more natural solution is supplementing with vitamins B6 and B3, which allow your body to conserve the amino acid tryptophan and convert that tryptophan into serotonin.

Vitamin B12 and other B vitamins play a role in producing brain chemicals that affect mood and other brain functions. Low levels of B12 or B6 may be linked to depression. The Rotterdam Study, conducted in 2002, supports this suggestion. Of nearly four thousand elderly people who participated, researchers found that many of those who had depressive symptoms also had vitamin B deficiencies.[43]

Vitamin D

Vitamin D, which we get from the sun and certain foods, is a truly remarkable vitamin our bodies historically need to function properly. It is an essential fat-soluble nutrient that helps keep bones healthy and strong, aids cell growth, and boosts immune function. There has been research examining the relationship of vitamin D to seasonal affective disorder (SAD), schizophrenia, and depression.

In a prospective birth study, vitamin D supplements were administered in the first year of life. In this clinical trial, it was noted that an intake of 2,000 IU of vitamin D or more per day was associated with a reduced risk of developing schizophrenia later on in life.[44]

In a cross sectional study of eighty older participants, more than half were noted to have vitamin D levels that were abnormally low. The lower the levels of vitamin D, the more likely they were to have Alzheimer's and clinically significant symptoms of depression.[45]

5-HTP

Commonly used for sleep disorders, 5-HTP (5-Hydroxytryptophan) can help insomnia, depression, anxiety, migraine and tension-type headaches, fibromyalgia, obesity, premenstrual syndrome (PMS), premenstrual dysphoric disorder (PMDD), attention deficit-hyperactivity disorder (ADHD), seizure disorder, and Parkinson's disease. 5-HTP is a chemical by-product of the protein building block L-tryptophan and is also produced commercially from the seeds of an African plant known as *Griffonia simplicifolia*.

5-HTP works by increasing the production of the chemical serotonin in the brain. Serotonin can affect sleep, appetite, temperature, sexual behavior, and pain sensation. When 5-HTP increases the synthesis of serotonin, it can be positively used for several diseases where serotonin is believed to play an important role, including depression, insomnia, obesity, and many other conditions, side-effect free. It is also safe for children and studies have shown promising results when used for night terrors and ADHD in kids and teens.[46]

St. John's Wort

St. John's wort is a flowering herb that has been used for centuries for medicinal purposes, including to treat mild to moderate depression. If you've heard that you should not take St. John's wort with specific drugs, this is not likely because of any adverse reactions between drugs and the herb. Instead, it is because the herb propels ALL chemicals in your body to work at maximum efficiency, including any drugs you are currently taking. In other words, St. John's wort makes anything you put into your system more powerful.

A Cochrane Collaboration review on St. John's wort concluded that the herb has superior efficacy to placebos in treating depression and is as effective as standard antidepressant pharmaceuticals for treating depression, with fewer adverse effects than pharmaceuticals. St. John's wort has additionally been proven to treat addiction, alcoholism, anxiety, OCD, HIV/AIDS, hepatitis C, and inflammation, as well as muscle pain, nerve disorders, menopause, chronic fatigue syndrome, and more! The uses for St. John's wort are endless, carry fewer effects than Rx drugs, and are completely healthy for you![47]

Nature's Anxiety Fighters

Antianxiety medications are some of the most commonly prescribed medications in the United States. They also carry some of the scariest real effects! You'll find that these drugs have negatively affected patients in study after study, instead of addressing the true causes of anxiety.

Anxiety is defined by a fear or nervousness about what might occur, while stress is described as a physical, mental, or emotional strain or tension. Roughly 7.3 percent of the population suffers from an anxiety disorder categorized by extreme anxiety that is seriously inhibiting and can affect how the sufferer thinks, feels, and acts.

Regardless of which one plagues you, each of us faces emotional turmoil resulting from stress on occasion. This can get us down temporarily, or it can be a huge roadblock to accomplishing our dreams or even enjoying our normal day-to-day activities! Clinical anxiety is the most common mental illness in the United States, affecting forty million adults in the country.

There are many theories as to why anxiety occurs, such as financial stress, health concerns, or hormonal changes. Many proactive alternatives to pills exist that will truly help you against your battle with stress and anxious feelings! Nature has a cure for anxiety. Below are a few of the most powerful natural alternatives. You need only take a dropper full of tincture or a tablespoon of spice to experience incredible anxiety and stress relief. As mentioned earlier, always consult with your naturopath, a doctor, and an online source about any interactions between certain spices, herbs, and drugs. These natural antianxiety remedies provide relief in minutes to hours. I know lifelong insomniacs who've received their first real, uninterrupted sleep EVER after just one cup of valerian tea before bedtime. (I also experienced this benefit the very first time I tried it!) Along with many of the meditation exercises mentioned previously, these natural remedies are an incredible way to take back your health and your power. You can find more natural anxiety relief options and keep up with my new finds at www.theorganiclifeblog. com/noanxiety.

∽∽∽∽

ANTIANXIETY MEDICATIONS AND THEIR SIDE EFFECTS

Commonly Prescribed Antianxiety Medications:

Xanax, Valium, Klonopin, Ativan, Serax, Librium, Norpramin, Elavil, Trazodone, Lexapro, Effexor, Cymbalta, BuSpar, Depakote, Lyrica, Neurontin, Ambien

Common Side Effects from Antianxiety Medications:

Fatigue, memory loss, nausea, blurred/double vision, disorientation, confusion, sleepiness, cold hands, weakness, dizziness, increased anxiety, slow reflexes, brain fog, slurred speech, poor coordination, stomach upset, addiction, sleep-driving, headache, sleepwalking, pounding heart, sweating, long-term cognitive impairment, hallucinations, depression, amnesia, abnormal behavior, withdrawal reactions, suicidal behavior, violence, homicidal ideation, increased hostility

Natural Anxiety Fighters

Magnesium

Magnesium is nature's original chill pill. Several studies have looked at how stress levels affect this common mineral in the body.[48] They found that during periods of extreme stress, magnesium is often used up a lot by our bodies. This suggests a common link between magnesium deficiency and anxiety. When a person experiences an anxiety attack, it may be because they are magnesium deficient.

In fact, it seems that a significant portion of the country is magnesium deficient, potentially leading to mass anxiety. On top of this, we may also be using up our magnesium reserves as a result of our anxiety, thus contributing to more anxiety, more stress, and feeding a never-ending cycle and negative "body loop."

Magnesium is known to play a crucial role in over seven hundred metabolic processes in the human body. It helps to regulate the nervous system by protecting your heart and arteries, which are important for anyone experiencing regular anxiety. To cure your anxiety, you'll ideally want your heart rate to be as low as possible. Magnesium supports this.

Magnesium is available in supplement form as a powder or capsule. I recommend the powder as it can be added with diversity and ease. You can add magnesium powder to your drinks or meals throughout the day to contribute to a stress-free, manageable life. Magnesium is easily dissolvable, making it perfect for adding to calming teas, baked goods or water. Foods high in magnesium include avocado, kelp, brown rice, cashews, parsley, and soybeans. When you find yourself craving these foods, it means you are low on magnesium and need to stock up! Bonus: these foods make an incredibly delicious, magnesium-rich salad; simply mix them all together in a bowl!

Melatonin

Melatonin is found in all known life-forms, including animals, plants, fungi, and bacteria. In humans it is produced in darkness, usually at night, by the pineal gland, a small endocrine gland located in the center of the brain but outside the blood–brain barrier. It is known as the "time-keeping hormone" because of the effects it has on balancing out our circadian rhythms. When we have circadian rhythm disorders, we can suffer from severe insomnia, or lack of sleep. This leads to severe mood changes, lack of inhibitions, stress, and anxiety.

We produce the most melatonin in our life at around four months of age. That is assuming that we've received proper nutrition, sleep, and care during this time. Even the care we receive by our mother when we're still in the womb is crucial to our melatonin production. After the first four months of life, we need to replenish melatonin ourselves. As we age, we continue to lose our melatonin production.

By prompting a stronger immune system, melatonin paves the way for essential nutrients to be diverted to the healing of the nerves. You can take capsules by mouth before bed to experience maximum results. Additionally, melatonin has also been shown to be effective for withdrawal from drugs such as Valium and Xanax. Also, look out for skincare products with melatonin in them: this "time-keeping hormone" has been proven in multiple studies to tackle fine lines and reverse wrinkles. I use it as the main ingredient in my organic beauty line, Genetix, specifically for this purpose. It may be your supplemental and topical fountain of youth.

Valerian

Popular throughout Europe and the United States, where it grows abundantly, valerian root contains a number of active chemical compounds. These include different alkaloids, but the most important may be gamma-aminobutyric acid, or GABA (mentioned above, in ways to fight depression), which is vital for brain function and helps to inhibit the stress-causing neurotransmitters that can lead to a lack of sleep or persistent anxiety.

This is the same active compound that is triggered by Valium, but valerian is a far safer and milder alternative to this addictive drug.[49] This fact has been backed up by clinical research in the past few decades,[50] but the herb's history goes much further back. Valerian has been used as a medicinal herb since at least the time of ancient Greece and Rome. Hippocrates described its properties, and Galen prescribed it as a remedy for restlessness and insomnia. In the sixteenth century valerian tea was prescribed for sick women.

As well as being an effective sleep aid and antianxiety remedy, valerian is also used for abdominal cramps, nervousness, obsessive thoughts, muscle relaxation, and insomnia.

To prepare valerian tea, take one bag per cup of hot water and allow it to steep for approximately ten minutes. When using valerian tea for insomnia or to get a better night of rest, drink it at night before bed in order to achieve the best results. I also recommend drinking this tea regularly, since it may take more than one night before taking a prominent effect. You can also take it as a tincture or supplemental capsules.

Passionflower

In 1569 Spanish explorers discovered passionflower in Peru and named it so because they believed the flowers symbolized Christ's passion and his approval for their explorative spirits. They used it as a sedative as well as for calming nerves.

A single dose of passionflower has been proven to decrease anxiety in patients who are about to undergo surgery. Additionally, another clinical trial found that passionflower is just as effective as benzodiazepines like Valium or Xanax for generalized anxiety disorder.[51] In this study, 36 individuals with generalized anxiety disorder compared passionflower to the standard antianxiety drug Oxazepam. Half the patients received 45 drops a day of a liquid passionflower extract; the other subjects received 30 milligrams of Oxazepam. Conclusion: Both treatments were equally effective by the end of the trial. However, passionflower was superior in terms of carrying no side effects. Oxazepam caused many job-related problems such as daytime drowsiness.

Ariel's WILD Habit Cured Her Stress

Ariel was a lot like that one friend we have. You know the one. She's always manicured, fashionable, and, most noticeably, she's always *stressed*. Always running from one meeting, event, and party to the next. Ariel was living off of panic and Valium. She'd start her day with three cups of coffee without blinking an eye. On her way to work, a popular energy drink became her go-to, so she could whiz through a twelve-hour day before heading on one of three grueling subway trains back home. Once Ariel was through her apartment doors, she ingested her Valium and collapsed into bed, relying exclusively on this pharmaceutical drug to put her to rest.

Ariel was sick of this cycle. She felt, looked, and acted like crap—to herself as well as to her friends, family, and colleagues. Her work, relationships, and body image were all suffering. Her health was declining, and she knew she needed a change.

After making this commitment, Ariel knew that the first thing she had to change was her habits. That night, Ariel started the process by simply preparing herself a tea. This tea contained valerian root, hot water, organic honey, and ice. Ariel let the drink infuse in her fridge overnight. In the morning, instead of her usual coffee, she instead began by taking a GABA supplement with ice cold lemon water. This refreshed her skin, detoxified her body, and set her mind in motion for having a great day. Ariel then grabbed the valerian iced tea and sipped it on her way to work. She drank it as necessary throughout the day.

On day one, not only was Ariel not fighting the morning jitters, but by noon she began to feel much calmer overall. A sense of well-being began to take over, and Ariel found herself ending her workday early for the first time in a long time. She walked down to the Hudson River and took a leisurely stroll before getting on her train home after rush hour. She opened a book, put on headphones, and listened to a meditation track—for the first time ever.

Ariel has practiced these new WILD habits for over a year and a half now—to immense benefits! Each night she prepares herself a valerian tea, each afternoon she takes a stroll down the Hudson, and every day she reads a different, new, and interesting page in a book and practices her meditation. Her friends, family, and colleagues have all noticed this change for the better. Even though she works fewer hours, Ariel has been able to get more done, and she received a promotion last year. Most miraculously, Ariel no longer needs to rely on Valium to put her to sleep at night. A double dose of her valerian iced tea before bed has done the trick for almost two years.

Ariel recently got engaged to a man she met around the time of this radical shift, a chance encounter she chocks up to her new WILD habit. She and her soulmate met on the train—the one Ariel used to always miss while she was slaving away at work.

ഝഝഝഝ

There are many natural ways to treat depression, anxiety, and sleep disorders that have proven success rates and no dangerous side effects. They are worth investigating if you find you have mild symptoms of depression or anxiety or if you would like to try to wean off of prescription medications (with your doctor's guidance) and supplement with natural alternatives to see which work best for you. Besides the more serious diagnoses like physical pain or mental health issues, nature can also provide remedies for common skin conditions, as we'll see in the next chapter.

CHAPTER ELEVEN

Green Beauty for Glowing Skin

Toxicity shows up for us in a lot of ways. It remained hidden in our food for decades and has been lurking in our beauty products for almost a century. I once learned that my skin enemy was hard water—and coming from my own faucet every time I took a bath or shower! You may have heard that even your cleaning products aren't truly clean. Where does it end?

By the time I started to address my own inner glow, I was at my wits' end with my skin. I faced large, red bumps that were impossible to conceal all over my face. Psoriasis plagued me on my legs and arms. Dry skin stung. Painful cystic acne popped up not just on my face but basically anywhere it felt like. Every week I was faced with a new set of tender red bumps all over my neck, back, thighs, and other sporadic parts of my body. It didn't feel like me and it didn't look like me. It hurt every time I moved my jaw, a painful and embarrassing reminder that I had cystic boils along my jawline.

I was desperate to solve my skin issues. One problem: I had already tried everything a dermatologist can recommend. I had been back and forth to dermatologists, estheticians and so-called skin experts since I was eleven years old.

I'd tried everything including Minocycline and Accutane as well as gels, creams, steroids, birth control, Proactiv, facials, diet changes, visiting expensive dermatologists, giving up dairy products—you name it! They had all left me depressed and dismayed. With skin that looked rough, bumpy, dehydrated, and was showing early signs of aging and traces of the long, late nights I'd spent working in college, a few years ago I walked into my modeling agency in LA and was blatantly told by my agent that I had to clean up my skin—or consider another career.

It stung to hear this, and I had no idea where to start. I had no budget for beauty and no background in glamour. I did know one thing: ingredients that were good for my skin and ingredients that weren't. As a scientist, I also knew most basic chemical compound names. So imagine my surprise when I turned around the bottles of some of the most widely recommended products before purchasing them. I was astounded. What faced me was a daunting list of unpronounceable ingredients—not ingredients that were known to heal skin, but chemicals! LOADS of them! Chemicals, fragrances, and toxic garbage. What the hell?! *Why was there formaldehyde in my shampoo?! Why was my bodywash made with harsh sulfates? How did PEGs, which have been found in breast cancer tumors, end up in my deodorant?!* Was this what I had been washing my hair with and brushing my teeth with and soaking my body in every day of my life?! How could this be?

I was about to learn that I was facing more than just troubled skin. I was facing a beauty industry that was built on a few major falsehoods about the proper ways of treating and taking care of ourselves. With only a few days of research and a steel resolve to find out the real origin of my severe skin conditions, my skin and my mind were forever changed. If you suffer from frustrating skin problems, this chapter will offer natural, nontoxic solutions to help your skin heal and glow.

Solving Our Skin Problems

Your skin is the largest and most important organ in your body, as it's your front line of defense. Male or female, don't be fooled into thinking this doesn't apply to you. People notice your skin. It's the one thing you can't hide. And when you suffer from skin conditions like psoriasis, eczema, or cystic acne, it can be frustrating and downright embarrassing, especially when a flare-up occurs right before a hot new date or an important meeting at work.

Today, I finally have the skin I always dreamed of having. Going from painful bumps every day and uncontrollable breakouts to an even, toned, clear complexion is my not-so-small health miracle. I wake up to glowing, freckled, dewy, beautiful, refreshed skin! I could not be happier with my complexion, and the confidence I've gained with clear skin has allowed me to do things I used to only dream of doing. I used to be afraid to go out, to talk to people, to have in-person meetings, to make videos, to meet new people . . . you name it! This held me back in unimaginable ways. My new, natural skin practices have given me my life back.

Besides seeing a dermatologist when it was "bad," I straight up ignored my skin for twenty-five years. I was pretty ignorant about beauty in general. For instance, I didn't know about moisturizing and toning (we'll cover these soon—don't worry!) Now, skincare is basically my top self-care ritual. I absolutely love using organic potions, Eastern beauty techniques, and natural products to achieve a tip-top glow and clear skin. I've found supplements that completely cured my cystic acne and psoriasis, I've experimented with green products that have seriously reversed the aging process, and I've indulged in spa-quality, at-home rituals that rival the effects of Botox. I truly care for my skin from the inside out, using many of the methods mentioned in this chapter.

Here is how I got rid of my cystic acne and solved my skin problems for good. . . .

Soft Water

You'll know you have hard water in your shower if you experience any of these symptoms after showering: dry skin, itchiness, flakiness, increased skin inflammation, filminess, or dry hair and scalp. Hard water is high in alkaline (pH) and also contains high levels of minerals like magnesium, calcium, and iron. This clogs and irritates your skin.

Hard water had done a number on my skin, but it took me months to identify this as one of the main culprits! The remedy is switching to a water filter for your showerhead. Soft water helps your body clear toxins, fight infections, and oh yeah—it won't take ten minutes to wash product out of your hair!

You can check if you have hard water in your area (and pick up an affordable remedy!) at www.theorganiclifeblog.com/hardwater.

Healing Tea

Want to know the world's most consumed psychoactive drug? Nope, it's not acid, mushrooms, cocaine, or marijuana. It's probably not what you think. . . .

It's caffeine.

The beverage most of us rely on every day to wake up—coffee—may be doing a number on your skin! Caffeine is a stimulant drug that (when ingested) can cause disruption to your gut, which is where the start of your clear skin truly begins. Caffeine also messes with your hormones, namely your stress hormone and your adrenal glands, which is a huge disruption to your oil production.

On top of that, it's a diuretic, adding a super dehydrating effect that I think we can all agree we'd like to skip. But don't worry, you can literally drink your way to amazing skin! Try replacing coffee with teas specifically designed to help you wean off. Teeccino, a substitute tea made with barley and flavored to taste like coffee, is one of my favorites. Or just make your own drink at home with some fresh herbs like mint, cacao, or lavender flowers and warm milk, cinnamon, honey, and turmeric.

Make sure you're choosing teas that are full of healing herbs and flowers like hibiscus, chamomile, mint, basil, or berries. These all contain flavonoids that are incredible for skin health. You truly want your glow to come from the inside—out!

Olive Leaf

I was introduced to olive leaf when I asked my family how the man I know as Dad, my grandfather (who is 100 percent Irish!), had such dark, illuminated, golden skin—year round. There was a story: Supposedly he was born prematurely and very sick. After he was born, a 1930s doctor in Ireland wrapped him in olive leaves to starve out the sickness for the first six months of his life. Other than a few brief moments to feed and get changed, he was rarely unwrapped from the olive leaves. Over time the olive leaf changed his skin color to a golden tan, which stuck for life. I know. I'm kind of jealous, too. I was also intrigued and started my research immediately. It turns out this story may be based in truth!

Olive leaves and olive leaf extract—both from the leaves of the olive tree rather than the fruit—also have many health benefits, including the potential to boost the immune system and to fight off harmful bacteria. Clinical trials have shown olive leaf extract as having potential in the treatment of viral diseases like herpes, pneumonia, and even the flu. Pop some supplements if you feel ANY sickness coming on!

Olive leaf is also known as "liquid gold." Wounds heal faster with olive leaf extract. According to a study published in a 2011 issue of *Journal of Medicinal Foods,* wounds treated with olive leaf extract showed 87 percent increased closure and 35 percent better strength compared to wounds treated with a commercial ointment.[52]

How does it work so well? Oleuropein, a type of secoiridoid and one of the active ingredient in olive leaf, is a powerful component to its healing methods. Many studies have confirmed it as an antioxidant, antimicrobial, and anti-inflammatory compound. Olive leaf contains linoleic acid, a fatty acid that helps moisturize and keep moisture from evaporating from skin. Because of its unique ability to mix with water, it helps your skin drink in the moisture without clogging pores. Oleuropein extract of olive leaf reduced reddening of the skin, dehydration, and blood flow to the skin better than vitamin E, according to a study published in a 2008 article in *International Journal of Cosmetic Science.*[53]

This makes it a great hydrator for all types of skin, even sensitive and combination skin that may be prone to acne. Personally, olive leaf also helps me to maintain a tan (I fight anemia, as mentioned in Chapter 8, and this helps so much!), and it brings a glow to my skin that I just love. It's a powerful anti-wrinkle fighter, too. You can consume it as a supplement and use olive oil or olive oil-based products as an oil cleanser.

Vitamins and Supplements

The reason that most conventional treatments for acne and skin issues don't work is that they fail to treat the real issue: your insides. Steroids, antibiotics, and even heavy-duty prescription medications skip over the one thing that truly does need to change for your new, clear skin to stick—your body needs to be in balance.

It wouldn't be an exaggeration to say that supplements have completely saved my skin in a variety of ways and on many levels. If you're frustrated with dry skin, cracked lips, acne, eczema, or a dull complexion, a supplement is most likely your answer! Many supplements have the power to give you a younger look, a natural tan, and clear skin if consumed every day or at least a few times per week. One of the top questions I receive is what supplement companies you can trust. You can find my current favorites and recommendations at theorganiclifeblog.com/skinsupplements. You can start by taking one at a time and slowly incorporate as many as you need to treat your skin problems directly.

FENUGREEK

Fenugreek has a high concentration of vitamin B1, which is responsible for generating energy from food. With this vitamin you can maintain healthy skin, hair, and nails. Fenugreek is a rich source of vitamin K, which is why you will inevitably find it in various skincare creams.

Doctors also use vitamin K as it helps in blood clotting. Assorted properties in vitamin K help to treat stretch marks and spider veins, fade scars, and reduce dark circles, and fenugreek is one of the richest sources of it. Other minerals in fenugreek like calcium, magnesium, zinc, selenium, and iron help to treat minor to moderate skin problems.

ECHINACEA

This supplement smells like honey and has a myriad of skin benefits; it is often used in antiaging serums, moisturizing lotions, and skin refreshers. Echinacea extract works like magic on your face. It soothes the skin by bringing down the swelling of the skin tissues, including inflammation that can cause acne, eczema, and psoriasis. It also helps fight acne-causing bacteria and provides freedom from acne in the long run. Rich in tannins, this substance works like an astringent and has a shrinking effect on skin cells. When used over time, it helps in reducing the appearance of wrinkles by up to 55 percent.

Rhodiola rosea

Rhodiola is probably most well-known for its ability as an adaptogen used for reducing stress and its negative effects. But that's not all it does. This herb can also be successfully used to restore the skin and bring back its youthful look. *Rhodiola* contains powerful anti-oxidants that can remove toxins and free radicals from the body.

Toxins and free radicals are not only dangerous to our health but also very damaging to the skin, making us look old before our time. Studies have shown that *Rhodiola* is comparable to vitamin C as an antioxidant, and you probably know how effective vitamin C can be for the skin! You can get *Rhodiola* in supplement form at your local grocery store or pharmacy.

Vitamin C

Okay, maybe you didn't know how beneficial vitamin C was for your skin . . . *now you will!* Vitamin C plays an important role in cellular synthesis, helping your body to produce collagen and preventing UV damage and the toxic effects of pollutants like cigarette smoke and overexposure to sunrays. Aging causes a steep decline in vitamin C content of the skin, so the older we get, the more important it is to supplement with vitamin C. Vitamin C can be applied topically to the skin or taken as a tincture or supplement once daily.

DIM

Who knew that the true key to curing my hormonal skin issues—especially my cystic acne—for good was getting passed by every time I went to the pharmacy (ironically, for a new skin Rx)? The last thing I was missing was supplements, which have truly been the big game changer for me.

Diindolylmethane (DIM) acts as an estrogen regulator. It balances the estrogen in your body, straightening out your hormones and allowing your skin to stop completely freaking out. It's become one of my personal favorites and has been one of the most useful herbs for curing hormonal skin issues for my friends, family, and clients. Those with hormonal acne or hormonal imbalances associated with menstruation, PMS, perimenopause, menopause, or postmenopause may benefit immensely from this supplement, as it balances hormones, supports "good estrogen," gets rid of "bad estrogen," and can even be a substitute for HRT (hormone replacement therapy)! I've known dozens of women who've seen drastic, overnight improvements in their skin with this one supplement. Although the bottle may recommend two doses per day, I see really incredible results when I take four DIM Plus capsules from Nature's Way per day, especially right before I experience PMS or PMDD.

I woke up the first week of taking DIM completely acne free! After years of trying absolutely everything to solve my skin issues, this was no small miracle. If I miss my DIM supplements, I do see the same symptoms that I used to have. Bumps pop up. Pores get clogged. Cysts form. Not pretty. If I take my DIM supplements, I don't ever have to worry—not even about a small blemish around that time of the month. My pores shrink, my oil is controlled, my T-zone is less shiny, and my skin is smoother.

Green Beauty Tips

Cheap, pharmacy products were all I ever bought before I switched to green beauty. And I'm actually glad I never invested too much into makeup or conventional beauty products before, because the expensive stuff doesn't work much better—unless it's made naturally! Conventional skin care is full of toxins and nasties that your skin hates, such as harsh SLS, parabens, dyes, parfum, and fragrances.

If you've tried everything but are still seeing skin issues, switch to a brand that only uses organic, natural oils and herbs in their products. If you see anything you can't pronounce or wouldn't eat, don't buy it and don't put it on your body! Our skin absorbs close to 100 percent of what we put on it.

Also, skip alcohol-based toning for a few dabs of apple cider vinegar on a cotton pad in the morning, and drink plenty of water throughout the day.

Masks

Anyone who truly knows me knows that I love a good green beauty mask. A thoughtfully made face mask works to simultaneously exfoliate and moisturize your skin. Masks work to pull out deep lurking bacteria from the skin, giving you a glowing visage that you'll be proud to show off. You'll start to love touching and showing off your face—no makeup needed! Incorporate an organic mask into your skin routine two to three times a week for the best results. My favorite DIY mask, which was recently featured by *Forbes*, goes a little something like this:

The *Forbes* Face Mask

INGREDIENTS:

1 tablespoon olive oil
1 teaspoon activated charcoal
1 tablespoon zinc
1 tablespoon cinnamon
1 tablespoon baking soda
1 tablespoon nutmeg
1 tablespoon salt
1 tablespoon cacao

1. Combine ingredients in a small bowl. Mix together thoroughly with a wooden spoon.

2. Add water a little at a time and mix thoroughly until it is a muddy consistency.

3. Apply to face, neck, and décolletage using a fan or makeup brush. Allow to dry on skin for 10 to 15 minutes, but remove while still damp.

Voila! A perfect complexion is yours! You can purchase all of these ingredients on Amazon or at your local health food store.

Toners

Toning remains one of my favorite beauty rituals, and it's one of my best kept secrets to achieving glowing skin and a toned, even complexion. If you're doing everything you can to try to achieve your dream complexion and still falling short, incorporate toning into your skincare routine every day. It should be considered an important part of the cleansing process. A good toner will remove any remaining bits of oil, dirt, and debris left behind by the cleanser.

More important, toner will help soothe, nourish, and hydrate the skin while restoring its delicate pH balance. Toning can be done throughout the day, in the morning, and at night. There are two important ways to tone, and you should practice each ritual at least once a day. One method is to spray a cotton cloth or ball with your toner and cleanse your face. The other method is to spritz your toner generously over your face. You can even do this after applying makeup for a dewy, fresh glow.

My favorite toner is simple and easy to make. Ready? It's a spray bottle of fresh, filtered, soft water and ten drops of organic rose essential oil. That's *it*. Rose water has anti-inflammatory properties that can help reduce the redness of irritated skin as well as reduce the frequency and appearance of acne, dermatitis, and eczema. It's also relaxing, aromatic, and refreshing.

Oils and Serums

Applying face oils and serums should be part of your everyday skincare routine. There's a reason these thicker liquids have been used since ancient times from head to toe. These healthy oils infuse your skin with potent botanicals and nourishing ingredients, and they can clear everything from acne to wrinkles to emotional or environmental damage. You can use them on your face and body to achieve a dewy, hydrated complexion. While you're drying off after a shower or bath, pat your skin dry rather than rubbing it, and leave a little water on the skin. Lock in the moisture by applying an organic body oil, or just use plain olive, grapeseed, or coconut oil from your kitchen. Avoid using coconut oil on your face if you have acne-prone skin, and don't use it as a moisturizer either, because the rich fats in coconut oil can clog pores. An alternative like argan oil or vitamin E oil might be better suited for your skincare needs.

Even if you already have an oily complexion, you can find the oil you should be using. There is an amazing collection of all-natural and organic skin-care brands that can help you on your journey to healthy, clear, beautiful skin. I was inspired to invent three serums that address sensitive, troubled, and aging skin: Genetix Detox Repair Serum for acne-prone skin, Glow Brightening Serum for troubled or dull skin, and Cellular Recovery Serum, an anti-aging youth serum. They're organic, melatonin-infused, herb and vitamin-enriched serums that support and heal the skin. I am constantly updating information about the current and best organic products I use and adore over on The Organic Life blog.

Moisturizers

Moisturizers are your final step in keeping your skin balanced and hydrated. They lock in all the hard work we did masking, toning, and using our oils and face serums. If your skin gets dehydrated, dry, or it looks dull and wrinkles appear, you may be lacking in this crucial skin-care step. You may see flakiness, and your makeup will not go on evenly. Moisturizer keeps your skin looking and feeling soft and supple.

You should use moisturizer no matter what your skin type is, be it dry, oily, combination, or normal. It's best to get a moisturizer with natural SPF (zinc) to help protect from the external environment, but some moisturizers, like those with cocoa, vitamin E, and shea butter, have natural sun protection. Apply moisturizer to your whole body, especially after a shower or bath. Some of my favorite organic moisturizers are by Pai Skincare, Odacite, and Metta Skincare. You can keep up with my current favorites over at www.theorganiclifeblog.com/faces.

FIVE WILD HABITS FOR GLOWING SKIN

1. Cut out caffeine and alcohol, especially hard alcohol. They are dehydrating to the body and skin. You'll notice an instant brightening to your skin if you cut back a little bit, and you'll achieve a year-round, gorgeous glow by cutting them out completely.

2. Take inventory of the products you're currently using. These seemingly innocent culprits can cause our bodies to produce inflammatory responses that irritate and inflame our skin.

3. If you can, replace your chemical-laden products with green beauty products. When looking for ingredients, if you can't pronounce it or wouldn't eat it, don't put it on your skin.

4. Wash your face with an organic black charcoal soap, spritz your rose toner, and use an organic serum and moisturizer every day. Mask one to three times a week. These rituals help us keep our skin's pH in balance by cleansing and exfoliating as well as hydrating.

5. Replace antibacterial or Rx drugs or products you use for your skin with supplements such as DIM, vitamin D, olive leaf, and *Rhodiola*.

Natural remedies like herbs, vitamins, and supplements can heal our bodies from the inside out. Even if you don't suffer from a specific skin issue, you will notice an unbelievable glow once you start supplementing your skin care and using clean beauty products. Unfortunately, many beauty products are not regulated and contain toxic chemicals that are detrimental to our health, and many brands have adopted intentionally deceptive names to seem natural or trustworthy, so it is more important than ever that you truly read labels and find natural, organic brands you can trust. The concept of beauty has changed drastically over the years and so has the industry standard. But what never goes out of style is the ability to capture a room with your confidence. Give yourself your best chance to be your true, most beautiful, authentic self and have that reflected perfectly back to you in the mirror. So focus on your attributes, build your strengths, and believe in yourself. Remember that you are beautiful—inside and out!

WILD Growth and Success

I wake up in the same bed, facing the same corner of the same room I was in when I spoke to my grandfather, my adoptive dad, for the last time. Before I watched him pass away five months ago. It's a surreal feeling. To be staring at the same crack in the same corner of the same room as when I last heard his cracking voice. It feels like nothing has changed, and yet my whole world is completely different. Almost incomprehensibly, I've been dealing with some of the worst emotional pain in my life, more than three thousand miles away from my family and most of my friends. I take a deep breath and sit up. I know I have to change my energy.

I leave the house to head down to the beach, in search of healing. Honestly, I am feeling so deeply bereaved on the way there. My mind is cloudy. Life feels incredibly unfair. The thoughts of him slipping into a coma, of his last breath, of him in pain seem completely inescapable. As much as I try to replace them with thoughts of him running marathons, kicking the soccer ball around, taking Olympic-style dives into my aunt's swimming pool, I can't. Nothing sticks. His last few moments on this earth—struggling for breath, struggling to live, struggling to die—are all that's on my mind.

I finally make it down to Swami's Beach, where Yogananda wrote *Autobiography of a Yogi* and ushered Kriya yoga into Western culture. *Autobiography* had been one of the first books I read in New York while going through withdrawal. Yogananda had become like a friend; his works were my greatest mentor. I'd talk to him in my meditations. I'd practiced Yogananda's form of yoga, Kriya, while coming off my meds to remarkable and often miraculous results. One minute I would be violently vomiting, and within a minute of my Kriya yoga breathing, I would have the strength and power to gain control of my stomach spasms, breathe, or sit up for just as long as it would take me to grab a bucket or transfer myself to another room. Swami's Beach, where *Autobiography* was inspired and written, was the first place I headed to when I got off the plane after coming home to California, just days after my dad's funeral. It felt like a true sanctuary.

As I hike by the beach, staring as the ocean dances, uncontrollable tears begin to flow. I had a certain destination in mind when I left the house, but instead I hike another mile down to Self-Realization Fellowship Temple, past steep cliffs that border the roaring sea. Tropical shrubs proudly line the streets. Joggers dash by in blurs, surfers proudly carry their boards, and manicured moms push strollers as they all intersect leisurely through one another's paths. It's a gorgeous view and the day is crystal clear and brilliant. I am allowing myself to cry in front of strangers, because I can't help it.

There, in front of me, are two empty chairs overlooking the horizon. Although I make this walk nearly every day, I have never noticed them before. I take a seat in one of the chairs and stare. From this distance, the ocean carries a tranquil calm.

After I moved to California, no one was sure if I was going to stay, least of all me. Dad received his cancer diagnosis during my road trip out to California, while I was cruising along sacred spaces in Arizona. I waited for him to obtain the results from a series of tests to find out what we were really facing. We all held our breath.

The cancer diagnosis returned: "Rare; unknown. Stage four." He was given six months to live.

He surpassed the deadline of his original diagnosis, then doubled it. Finally, it was two years later, and Dad was on lots of medication but still alive and visiting the gym, booking trips, golfing, and otherwise living his life as if nothing terrible had happened.

As I gaze at the blanket of blue surf, I am thinking about Dad's last breath. I am thinking about Dad running his last marathon. I am thinking about Dad asking if I want ice cream. I am thinking about Dad driving me to high school, soccer practice, dance lessons, voice lessons, and piano. I am thinking about Dad's diagnosis, his chemotherapy, his kidney surgeries, his three brain surgeries, his radiation, how he became paralyzed, and the last thing he said to me.

He had so much life in him, and I am hysterically crying now because life seems incredibly unfair. *Why,* I ask, *do good people have to die? Why was he taken from us? From me? Why does everyone I love die?*

I close my eyes, take a deep breath, and hear a voice say: *How can you be sad? Everything has been given to you.*

I open my eyes and look around. But either the person who said it has left, or . . .

I sit with those words for a moment.

How can you be sad?

Everything has been given to you.

A wave of peace rushes over me and I stop wondering. I start to feel—I swear—like I am sitting there with my dad. Although tears are still flowing, I have to smile.

I know my dad has already given me everything and anything I could ever have wanted. He affected my life in the best way possible. He took me in when he didn't have to. He raised me like his own daughter. He gave me everything: security, comfort, education, and, most of all, a second chance at life. He taught me about hard work and the hard-earned dollar. He taught me about family, sacrifice, and love. He loved me in a way that people rarely receive love. Unconditionally.

He may be gone, but I am here. Right now.

A legacy.

I have to appreciate that.

The longer I remained in California, the more Dad would always ask me if I planned on staying. Not because he wanted me back in New York (after all, I was flying back home to visit, help out with treatment, and care for him every month). I know Dad would ask because he wanted to make sure that California was where my destiny was supposed to take me. Most important, he was checking in to make sure that things were working out.

That means that the best way that I can live now is to ensure that things *do* work out. And maybe I don't have him here to guide me (at least not in the way that I was used to), but I know he's helping me resolve the kinks of life in his own way. I've been given everything I need—and he gave it to me.

In that moment, sitting next to that empty chair and feeling my dad's presence with me, I give thanks. I give myself blessings for my good health, beating heart, new life education, strong will, WILD habits, and a host of other things for which I've become extraordinarily grateful. I even thank him for finally passing over, as I know that life takes its natural course for everyone, and losing him was teaching me a lot about my own selfishness.

Honestly, watching him suffer so much was one of my greatest fears. Watching him take his last painful, shallow, broken breath will remain with me forever. Losing him to cancer was one of the most devastating realities that I could imagine, and I still bravely swallow the truth of his absence each and every day.

But now I smile. I smile on days I never, ever thought I'd be capable of smiling. That alone means everything to me, because it means it wasn't all for nothing.

I am feeling better.

Everything Has Been Given To You

In that depressing, lost moment, my WILD habits had kicked in. I had the *willingness* to leave the house. I showed *love* for myself by doing something different, even when I didn't feel like it. My *intuition* had lead me down to the cliffs, and then another mile down to the bluffs, where I had found the chairs. Once I received the message that I was there to hear, I had the *discipline* to accept that message and form a new attitude: gratitude.

Everything had been given to me. I had a brand-new life from the one I was looking at just a few months ago. I could be dead a hundred times over. But I wasn't dead. I was here. And I owed it to my dad to make sure I did the most with every new breath that I'd been gifted. With that discipline always at the forefront of my mind, I've kept at my goals without fail and now wake up to a drastically empowered and secure life—far different from the life I used to face. In the time since I made that promise to myself, I received an email offering me my first book deal. I was able to write that work with no trouble at all and watched that little book baby skyrocket to number one.

I secured jobs alongside some of my greatest personal heroes and mentors. I've watched my work propel my life. I've picked up magazines and books with my name proudly printed in them. I've been featured by some of the most well-respected platforms in the world. I've spoken to crowds of people ten times the size of the parties that used to scare me into staying home. I've performed my music on some of the most recognized stages in the game. I've found my tribe—professionally, personally, and socially. I was able to secure this book deal as well, which allowed me to bring an even deeper message and awareness into the world through another work. I've accomplished all the things I'd want Dad to be proud of me for, and I continue to check goals off the list daily.

Everything has been given to me to *succeed*. It's been up to me to make the most of that.

Conquer the Self-Pity Habit

How many times have you heard someone say, "If so-and-so had only gone through what I had gone through, they wouldn't be so . . ." There are a lot of people whose main joy in life consists of comparison—a small comfort to bring a sense of triumph into their own lives. We all want to believe that our trials in life are harder than others' difficulties. It gives us a sense of importance, or entitlement.

Self-pity is one of the worst habits that we have. Self-pity steals our joy. It creeps in and makes allowances for our faults, places blame on others, hinders the success of our WILD habits, and robs us of our self-respect. Don't ever allow someone, or some event, to take your happiness away from you. It is better to have your conscience, your logic, your health, and your sense of well-being than to have the approval of people.

No one took anything away from me. In fact, it was quite the opposite. I truly feel that in having my dad in my life for the twenty-seven amazing years that I did, I was given an extraordinary gift. I miss my dad. A lot. That's the truth. Nothing can replace him, it still hurts, and I grieve in ways I never saw coming. But the bigger truth is he'd want me to be happy.

Grief is messy. Often, as time goes on, it feels messier, because the memories are getting farther away. Every day forward is another day further away from that person's presence in your life. But we need to appreciate every moment, for the moment. Living in the present will help you to remain focused on your transformation and dedicated to your new WILD habits.

The best view of all is what you see in others. Your health, your happiness, and your livelihood are all influenced by your mind.

There is a lot of happiness cultivated in small things: in gratitude, in noticing details, in stopping and remembering, and in focusing on your breath. There is happiness in listening and in appreciating what is right in front of you, *right now.*

I encourage you to find your happiness.

Overcoming Self-Sabotage

Self-sabotage is a nasty behavior that affects even the most successful of us—it is when our self-pity manifests into actions that actually hold us back from realizing our goals and harms us. Unfortunately, we aren't always aware that we are sabotaging ourselves. The effects of our behavior may not show up for some time, and other people may be hesitant to be honest with us about it. And, truthfully, connecting a behavior to a devastating consequence is still no guarantee we will change. However, it is possible to overcome almost any form of self-sabotage. People do it every day.

Self-judgment is the root of self-sabotage and it's a harmful habit. If you catch yourself judging, try replacing your negative thoughts with positive ones or asking your *higher self* for guidance. When you listen to your higher self, you're allowing your divinity to take the front seat. Your highest self is the most divine, perfect, true, intuitive part of you that knows how wonderful, perfect, and authentic you truly are—even if you're not embodying those traits at this moment. To connect to our higher self, we have to abandon our bad habits like self-judging and return to our WILD habits like self-love. Your highest self emerges when you consistently tap into the WILD Method to transform your life. Putting ourselves or others down is a classic self-judging technique. Changing your language is one of the most important things that you can do to stop yourself in your tracks.

For instance, if you're scared or hesitant about ending a relationship, instead of thinking, "I need to leave this person!" and feeling guilty or trapped, you may think "This person belongs in someone else's life" or "I deserve different and new, and this person does, too!" Leave yourself open to the idea that life goes on. You two truly may just not be right for one another.

For many people, admitting mistakes is difficult. You can only learn from your mistakes if you're willing to admit you've made them. As soon as you start blaming other people (or the universe itself), you've put a roadblock between yourself and your life lesson. Refusing to acknowledge your mistakes, or not acknowledging similar kinds of mistakes, is a refusal to acknowledge reality.

If you can't see the gaps, flaws, or weaknesses in your behavior, you'll always be trapped in the same behavior and limitations you've always had. When someone tells you you're being a baby, they might actually be onto something. Chances are, you're acting out behaviors you've carried with you your entire life—probably since you were a child!

Instead of dwelling on your mistakes, judging yourself, and ultimately engaging in self-sabotage, allow failure to be a lesson. Be courageous about changing your behavior and have the self-confidence to acknowledge where you went wrong. These things will, in themselves, make you feel better.

Nothing can hurt your self-esteem more than comparison—it's a harmful habit that many of us engage in. A lot of people set up situations for themselves where comparison is inevitable. They will actually place themselves in situations where they have no choice but to compare. They'll force others to compare them! Seem insane? It's common! I saw this all the time in my modeling career. Women will sit around for hours and do nothing BUT compare themselves to other women. They'll spend their time on internet envy gorging on their intense fixations. They'll buy the same clothes or wear the same things as others. Just to compare. This is a form of self-abuse.

I know it's tough, but you need to stop comparing yourself to other people. These comparisons are unfair because you don't know as much as you think you do about other people's lives, or what it's really like to be them. You don't know how curated their lives or personalities are. And it's not your job to worry about it. Just because someone earns a higher salary, lives in a beautiful home, or has a nicer car than you doesn't mean she has a better life. Besides, being perfect is exhausting. Being wild and free is fun. We are all unique and beautiful, and each of us has our own individual life purpose.

Be kind to yourself. Pay attention to each and every moment. Live your life with intention and do it carefully. Take pride in your actions. Take long baths, light candles, put on nice (natural!) perfume, or read some emails or texts from friends that make you happy. Remind yourself of what you're good at and go out into the world with a smile. The only person you should be competing against is yourself.

Self-victimization is a huge trigger for self-sabotage. All of those *"Why me?"* thoughts are doing **nothing** but taking blame from your own choices. Seeing a doctor about your "why me" thoughts does you no better. The growing tendency among many psychologists and medical practitioners is to classify all manner of behavioral problems as illnesses and diseases. When you receive a diagnosis, *what has changed?*

Psychotherapy sees many normal life events as trauma in need of healing, instead of as enriching experiences we can learn from. Taking responsibility for your own actions when you notice self-sabotage or self-victimization is not only the most important but also the ONLY step to truly changing your behavior—to eliminating your harmful habits and replacing them with WILD habits. Remember, a creator mentality is much more fulfilling than a victim mentality.

It truly is *ALL* about how you look at it!

Making the decision that you are unwilling to compromise your self-love behaviors for others is a really important step in making them last. You will not fear rejection or exhibit neediness when you learn to be true to yourself. When you are willing to take loving action on your own behalf—even if another person doesn't like it—you are truly alive. Losing people who don't love you for who you are means that you will gain people who want to be around you for EXACTLY who you are. Everyone wants to be around someone who is consistently striving to be someone better—someone like you!

Embrace Growth

One of the unhealthiest approaches to life is to make a decision that who you are is defined by a moment or period of time, after which you spend the rest of your life trying to still be that person. I had a friend (keyword: had) who just loved to point out to me how she was still the same person she'd been many years ago. She took great pleasure in saying things like, "You know me, Tara! I'm the same person I was when we met." This was completely reflected in my old friend's personality: She rarely learned from her mistakes, her relationships all seemed to fail, and she had no true sense of self. She put on the mask of whoever she was around, and her behavior was methodical and self-centered.

Look for people around you who proudly proclaim they are no different than they were the day they turned fifteen or twenty-two or thirty-six, or whenever. Do these people seem like flexible, easygoing, happy people? Often they are not. They are so busy insisting that nothing has changed for them that they're incapable of adopting new ideas, learning from others, or growing.

They may fully believe that they are "being themselves," but in reality they are often enslaved by the past and a particular image of themselves. Growth into every new age and stage of our lives is an essential part of being true to ourselves and to being emotionally healthy and whole. There is a healthy alternative: being someone who is still you, but who grows with the passing of each day and learns from her mistakes.

Decide that you will define yourself by what you are good at today, not by what you lack. Make a list of your strengths, your new WILD habits, and journal about things that made you proud of yourself during the course of the day. Also be careful about basing your self-worth on an older version of yourself. I used to be wonderful at playing the flute, for instance, but couldn't possibly call myself a flautist right now. That's okay. I've adjusted my beliefs about myself and what I AM currently good at doing. And I've motivated myself to be better at what I'm not so great at (yet!). Keep adjusting your self-image and your self-esteem to match your current abilities.

Allow yourself the space to become wiser than you were yesterday, and to proudly present that person to everyone you know. You can proclaim things out loud like, "I know I messed up last time, but this time I'm doing better." As you do this, you will literally feel a weight being lifted from your heart. I found that using this kind of language with yourself and your loved ones really cracks open relationships and leaves room for fresh, new things to grow, because it paves the way for forgiveness. Beautiful things grow in forgiveness. Forgiving past errors and working hard to make improvements on yourself with your new WILD habits is the key to unlocking the door to your happiness.

True Success

I had lofty dreams growing up. I wanted to open my own business, make music, and formulate skin-care products. I wanted to change people's lives. I wanted people to know who I was. I wanted to write for magazines, act in movies and music videos, and write best-selling books that would make people's lives better.

If you had told me ten years ago that I'd do even ONE of those things in the next decade, I wouldn't have believed you. If you told me seven years ago that I'd do them all in my first five years off prescription drugs, I would have laughed my ass off. You see, I didn't believe I was capable of much—either on drugs or off them. Drugs were the final answer. Stability, not success, was the goal.

I used to make the mistake of thinking that success was a *thing*. An accomplishment. A marriage. Your name on a book. Your book in a bookstore. True success is emotional success. True success feels like (at least for now) everything is done and right. It is a natural high, a way of life. True success is a lifestyle—a lifestyle full of WILD, healthy habits. Your happiness is your true success.

Successful people are not successful by accident. Success requires a lot of hard work, perseverance, learning, studying, sacrifice, and, most of all, love of what you are doing. And it's all worth it.

The Universe Is Always Listening

We all fight a duality of character. We have two sides: We possess a positive nature that wants us to help, love, and care, and a negative nature that surfaces when we are deeply hurt.

The universe is always listening. Quietly and intently. If you focus on the negative, you will receive more of it; if you focus on the positive—your dreams, goals, and WILD habits—that is what you will manifest into your life. Learning integrity and an ability to control your tendencies to blame or resent others will always help you to realize who you truly are. Every good thought we put out instead of a bad one really helps us in overcoming our personal battles and harmful habits.

Our negative nature wants to control our hurt or pain by blaming and resenting. Blame wastes emotional energy on resentment and anger. More importantly, it defeats the purpose of uncomfortable emotions. Uncomfortable emotions motivate behavior that will heal and improve. Blame makes you powerless to heal and improve. The ability to heal and improve reveals your true nature.

Alienation from our deepest values is a huge roadblock to figuring out our purpose. You cannot really be yourself unless you are true to the most important things to and about you. These will not be preferences or ego gratifications (as you would not want on your tombstone "She liked white wine" or "Here lies an insatiable ego"). The most important things to and about you as a person are your deepest values. Cultivating those and finding out why they give you pleasure is a true, fun part to becoming yourself.

I start by writing down things that make me happy to do, instead of a to-do list of projects that I need to finish. That normally refocuses me to figure out what's important to me and what truly makes me happy

The truth is, none of us are perfect (gasp! I know, right?).

We're all imperfect, growing, learning human beings. If you feel ashamed or insecure about any aspect of yourself and you feel that you have to hide those parts of you, whether physically or emotionally, then you have to come to terms with that. Learn to convert your so-called flaws into individualistic quirks that make you YOU. Don't beat yourself up, and avoid getting critical with yourself. We all get a blemish and have a bloat day and feel gross every now and again, sometimes for a lot longer than we should. Check yourself. Love yourself. Forgive yourself.

A common thing a lot of people do is copy others' actions. It seems like the best route to fit in, but really, shouldn't you want to stand out? Standing out is hard, yes, but that's what being yourself is all about. People have a real reverence for others who have a deep sense of themselves. Obtaining this deep sense of self is done by delving far and wide into who you know you are and what you're good at.

Whether it's your sense of style, your voice, or your character, explore it. Express yourself, learn to communicate, and watch the positive outcome. The universe always listens to your genuine, heartfelt requests. Turning your quirks into things people really enjoy will make you the best version of yourself possible!

Finding Your Heroes

Amelia Earhart, whose thirst for adventure made her the first female aviator to fly across the Atlantic Ocean, wrote in her journal that "adventure is worth it, in itself." Despite dozens of challenges, Sacagawea accompanied Lewis and Clark west with a newborn baby on her back and served as their guide. She even rescued Lewis and Clark's journals from a river during a rafting accident (the river is now named after her). Nellie Bly took off on a 25,000-mile adventure with nothing but the dress on her back, a heavy coat, a few pairs of underwear, and a small bag carrying her toiletries in 1889. There's also Laura Dekker, the fourteen-year-old girl who sailed around the world with nothing but her sailboat and her camera, just a few years ago (the must-watch documentary *Maidentrip* is on Netflix.)

These women had one thing in common: They did these things purely for fun. Because the sense of adventure made them happy.

They're some of my personal heroines, and they've helped inspire a courageous, happy-just-to-be-alive side of me that I will carry throughout my life. What is it about the carefree and fearless men and women before us that can propel our lives?

Personally, they've inspired me to become the globe-trotting, mountain-climbing, sunrise-surfing, jet-setting little business woman and boho love warrior I always wanted to be, and their lives have given me helpful and invaluable lessons that have opened my heart and mind to all of life's boundless possibilities. I better understand life's ultimate bounty of physical, mental, and emotional rewards.

Have you ever found yourself in a slump? Maybe you've faced your share of turmoil. Some of us agonize over whether or not we should go to a party or try our hand at a new career. We even question if we should cut or color our hair differently than last time, or if it's a good idea to drive to the grocery store!

All of this while digging deep down daily, fighting the ego and our harmful habits, and trying to figure out who we really are, why we're here, and what we're going to bring to the world. What footprints will we leave behind? Or maybe we're just trying to finish breakfast and get to work on time.

So how do we become the best, most fearless versions of ourselves? How do we elevate our vibration and ultimately our whole lives? What separates the greatest people in history from those who live with many ghosts—ghosts of things put off "for tomorrow" and never accomplished? How can we elevate our awareness, our salary, our passion, or our personal power? When you replace your harmful habits with your new WILD habits, you transform your life and open the door to living your passions and finding your purpose.

Find out what your heroes did. Read the autobiographies of some of the most famous and inspiring people who come to mind: Gandhi, Julie Andrews, Carrie Fisher, Malala Yousafzai, Carol Burnett, Dolly

Parton, Sheryl Sandberg, Drew Barrymore, Richard Branson, Johnny Cash, Dick Van Dyke, Shirley MacLaine, Priscilla Presley, Ozzy Osbourne, Benjamin Franklin, Mother Teresa, Lucille Ball, Barack Obama, and so many more—all have autobiographies they've written about their own lives! They are the best guidebooks in existence, as they contain some of life's greatest secrets, including how these successful people reached their goals. You can learn from their mistakes instead of making your own. When you can successfully avoid making the same mistakes that other people have made, this leaves you all the time in the world for creating a better, more empowering life for yourself.

Find Adventure in Everything

The number one question I get asked as an author is, "Tara, how do I start writing a book?"

My answer, every time?

"Just start."

The unknown is frightening, I get it. That blank page staring you in the face may be more intimidating than your grumpy boss on a Sunday afternoon. But getting started is the key to your future. Once you begin, things aren't so intimidating. They soon become part of a fun, thrilling adventure.

I know you've heard it before, but any life is really just what you make of it. That trip to the grocery store? Adventure. Writing that novel you always wanted to write? Adventure. Talking to that boy and getting a hot date? Adventure.

It doesn't matter if you travel the world, jump out of an airplane, or climb Mount Everest—if you don't think of it as an exciting adventure, it won't be. You'll be bored by it. Or worse, scared by it. So adopt the mentality that life is a big adventure, and life will surely act like it is!

Know Your Risks and Rewards

Risky action doesn't always have to be part of your everyday life, but it will get you out of the house. I used to have terrible social anxiety and would only go out if I either knew who was going to be there or—better yet—knew *no one* was going to be there. I ruined many possibly fun nights for myself by being afraid and self-conscious and never leaving my bed or dorm room.

If there's no risk, there's no adventure.

Think about if you knew what was going to happen every single moment for the rest of your life. There would be no point in living it! You'd get bored immediately. Risk is definitely part of the reward. So whether you're paddling out to surf for the first time, jumping off a high dive, taking a yoga class, or just leaving the house, find the risks you're comfortable with and let them grow into rewards. Rewards will nourish your soul. You'll give yourself the opportunity to have friendly, inspiring conversations, make interesting friends, and gain experiences that will change you for a lifetime.

Awaken Your Inner Child

Your inner child lives inside of you, and she has a voice. She still loves palm trees and coloring and Paris. He still enjoys trains and the walks in the park. A playful, comfortable spirit is totally essential to getting in touch with your happiest, most elevated self. You need to have fun as you go! If you're on a hike and you find yourself complaining or tired, stop, take a breath, and appreciate all the nature and clean air and trees and sights around you. Feel grateful for the ability to hike and the presence of mind to experience this moment.

And don't forget to do silly things! Jump in puddles and climb trees and swing on swing sets. It'll help you feel comfortable and grateful.

Sharing my adventures with my loved ones is one of my favorite parts of living in this day and age. Plus, it's free! The best, right? Adventure is the best education you'll ever have. You may learn more about yourself in one walk than you have in a decade. I invite my loved ones to come on walks and hikes with me, and I take my dogs everywhere I go. I feel as though I've learned unique lessons through nature that I can share with people, and I am always pleasantly surprised by what I hear back.

Finding Your Purpose

Many people find their passion, but miss their purpose. Your passion is your draw to a certain activity, and your purpose is the reason behind that draw. Maybe you always loved musical instruments, but you haven't ever figured out why. You're drawn to piano and finally, on a whim, sign up for piano classes at the local music store. After taking piano lessons for a few weeks, you start naturally tinkering around and then begin writing your own songs. This inspires you to start working on a full-length album. You finish it in a couple of energized months and put out music that people wind up absolutely loving. You feel ultimately fulfilled. Your passion was piano; your purpose was sharing your musical gift. If you go hard at something for a little while but you find yourself slacking after a week or two, it's probably not your passion or your purpose. Your passion and your purpose will be effortless. You can put it off for a little while, but in the end, it will be the one thing you cannot help but do.

Did you stop singing long ago but still hum tunes in the shower? Your purpose is music. Did you give up "cars" a long time ago but still tinker on your Honda every chance you get? Your purpose is mechanics. Maybe you never pursued a career in dance after your dance degree, but nothing brings you more joy than to twirl around in meadows every single spring. Your purpose is dance.

Having a meaning to your life is essential to continuing in a great direction, taming your harmful habits and turning them into WILD habits, and creating the kind of life you truly deserve. The spirit that will get you from scrambling around looking for the best version of you to automatically finding your true inner self has been within you all along. Define the choices you're making. This will ultimately help you to improve your life, your job, your friends, and your environment. Do this by consistently, consciously reminding yourself of how you've chosen to live, remember your destinations, plans, methods, and meaningful interests. Find something that personally fulfills you, and you will get up every single day with a smile on your face—and do it! This is sure to elevate your life and bring you closer to your true goal.

⁓⁓⁓⁓

I want to thank you for engaging with this book and empowering your life. I want to reach across whatever space and time may separate us and offer you my sincere blessings. May you have and accomplish whatever is truly important to you.

You don't have to search for a better life. That mission is over. Your new mission is simply to observe it, recognize it, embrace it, and be here—just where you are. The opportunity is right here, right now. Congratulations, my friend!

Have a WILD life.

Acknowledgments

There are so many people who made this book possible. I want to thank my incredible literary agent, Bill Gladstone, who has believed in me from moment one. I want to express gratitude to my amazing publishers and editors at SelectBooks, who took a chance on me and this body of work. I want to thank my out-of-this-world editors, Lara, Nancy, and Molly, who saw this book for what it could be and helped me make it so. Thank you to my incredible publicists at Sarah Hall Productions: Sarah, Lisa, Jessie, Carolyn, and Dana, who always know what I can become, even before I see it.

Thank you to my rescue pups, Raelie and Ruca, who sat by me for every page and made me smile whenever things got too serious. Thank you to my family. Thank you Mom, for letting me share your story in order to help others. I am so proud of you and I love you so much. Thank you Grandma, for everything—for raising me, for loving me, for helping me in so many ways. You will always have my heart.

Finally, thank you, Dad. Although you are no longer here on earth guiding me, I am keenly aware that you have helped me in ways both of this world and far beyond. I couldn't have done it without you.

Endnotes

1. Mao Shing Ni, "Live Longer with Pets," June 7, 2012, http://www.doctoroz.com/blog/mao-shing-ni-lac-dom-phd/live-longer-pets.

2. Lulu Chang, "Americans Spend an Alarming Amount of Time Checking Social Media on Their Phones," Digital Trends, June 13, 2015, https://www.digitaltrends.com/mobile/informate-report-social-media-smartphone-use.

3. Jean M. Twenge, "Have Smartphones Destroyed a Generation?" *The Atlantic,* September 2017, https://www.theatlantic.com/magazine/archive/2017/09/has-the-smartphone-destroyed-a-generation/534198.

4. Zoe Weiner, "7 Tips for Eliminating Toxic People from Your Life," *Mental Floss,* March 22, 2017, http://mentalfloss.com/article/93521/7-tips-eliminating-toxic-people-your-life.

5. Henry Ford, *My Life and Work: An Autobiography of Henry Ford* (New York: Classic House Books, 2009).

6. Remez Sasson, "How Many Thoughts Does Your Mind Think in One Hour?" accessed November 1, 2017, https://www.successconsciousness.com/blog/inner-peace/how-many-thoughts-does-your-mind-think-in-one-hour.

7. Raj Raghunathan, "How Negative Is Your 'Mental Chatter'?" *Psychology Today,* October 10, 2013, https://www.psychologytoday.com/blog/sapient-nature/201310/how-negative-is-your-mental-chatter.

8. Bill Moyers, *Healing and the Mind* (New York: Main Street Books, 1995).

9. John Whitman, *The Psychic Power of Plants* (New York: Signet, 1974), 52.

10. Roy F. Baumeister, Ellen Bratslavsky, Mark Muraven, and Dianne M. Tice, "Ego Depletion: Is the Active Self a Limited Resource?" *Journal of Personality and Social Psychology* 74.5 (1998): 1252-1265.

11. Vadim S. Rotenberg, "'Genes of Happiness and Well Being' in the Context of Search Activity Concept," *Activitas Nervosa Superior* 55.1-2 (2013): 1–14.

12. Ruut Veenhoven, "Healthy Happiness: Effects of Happiness on Physical Health and the Consequences for Preventive Health Care," *Journal of Happiness Studies* 9 (2008): 449–469.

13. S. L. Shapiro, J. A. Astin, S. R. Bishop, and M. Cordova, "Mindfulness-Based Stress Reduction for Health Care Professionals: Results From a Randomized Trial," *International Journal of Stress Management* 12.2 (2005): 164–176.

14. Daniel Goleman and Richard J. Davidson, *Altered Traits: Science Reveals How Meditation Changes Your Mind, Brain, and Body* (New York: Avery, 2017), 171.

15. "Effectiveness of a Meditation-Based Stress Reduction Program in the Treatment of Anxiety Disorders," *The American Journal of Psychiatry* 149.7 (1992): 936-943, https://doi.org/10.1176/ajp.149.7.936.

16. Daniel C. Cherkin, Karen J. Sherman, Benjamin H. Balderson, Andrea J. Cook, Melissa L. Anderson, Rene J. Hawkes, Kelly E. Hansen, and Judith A. Turner, "Effect of Mindfulness-Based Stress Reduction vs Cognitive Behavioral Therapy or Usual Care on Back Pain and Functional Limitations in Adults with Chronic Low Back Pain: A Randomized Clinical Trial," *JAMA: The Journal of the American Medical Association* 315.12 (2016): 1240-1249.

17. John T. Mitchell, Elizabeth M. McIntyre, Joseph S. English et al., "A Pilot Trial of Mindfulness Meditation Training for ADHD in Adulthood: Impact on Core Symptoms, Executive Functioning, and Emotion Dysregulation," *Journal of Attention Disorders* 21.13 (2017): 1105-1120, https://doi.org/10.1177/1087054713513328.

18. Richard J. Davidson and Antoine Lutz, "Buddha's Brain: Neuroplasticity and Meditation," *IEEE Signal Processing Magazine* 25.1 (2008): 176–174, https://www.ncbi.nlm.nih.gov/pmc/articles/PMC2944261.

19. J. Sanmukhani, V. Satodia, J. Trivedi, T. Patel, D. Tiwari, B. Panchal, A. Goel, and C. B. Tripathi, "Efficacy and Safety of Curcumin in Major Depressive Disorder: A Randomized Controlled Trial," *Phytotherapy Research* 28.4 (2014): 579-85, https://www.ncbi.nlm.nih.gov/pubmed/23832433.

20. Lauren Brown West-Rosenthal, "16 Foods That Stop Sugar," March 17, 2017, http://www.eatthis.com/stop-sugar-cravings.

21. J. S. Armstrong, "Mitochondrial Medicine: Pharmacological Targeting of Mitochondria in Disease," *British Journal of Pharmacology* 151.8 (2007): 1154-1165, http://doi.org/10.1038/sj.bjp.0707288.

22. C. Martijn et al., "Getting a Grip on Ourselves: Challenging Expectancies about Loss of Energy after Self-Control," *Social Cognition* 20.6 (2002): 441–460.

23. M. Gailliot et al., "Self-Control Relies on Glucose as a Limited Energy Source: Willpower Is More Than a Metaphor," *Journal of Personality and Social Psychology* 92.2 (2007): 325–336; M. Inzlicht and J. Gutsell, "Running on Empty: Neural Signals for Self-Control Failure," *Psychological Science* 18.11 (2007): 933–937; Baumeister et al., "The Strength Model of Self-Control," *Current Directions in Psychological Science* 16 (2007): 351–355.

24. Steven Greenberg and William H. Frishman, "Co-Enzyme Q10: A New Drug for Cardiovascular Disease," *The Journal of Clinical Pharmacology* 30.7 (July 1990): 596-608, http://dx.doi.org/10.1002/j.1552-4604.1990.tb01862.x; M. F. Beal, "Coenzyme Q10 Administration and Its Potential for Treatment of Neurodegenerative Diseases," *BioFactors* 9.2-4 (1999): 261-266, http://dx.doi.org/10.1002/biof.5520090222; K. Lockwood, S. Moesgaard, T. Hanioka, K. Folkers, "Apparent Partial Remission of Breast Cancer in 'High Risk' Patients Supplemented with Nutritional Antioxidants, Essential Fatty Acids, and Coenzyme Q10," *Molecular Aspects of Medicine* 15.1 (1994): s231-s240, https://doi.org/10.1016/0098-2997(94)90033-7; Franklin Rosenfeldt, Deborah Hilton, Salvatore Pepe, Henry Krum, "Systematic Review of Effect of Coenzyme Q10 in Physical Exercise, Hypertension, and Heart Failure," *BioFactors* 18.1-4 (2003): 91–100, http://dx.doi.org/10.1002/biof.5520180211.

25. A. J. Redig and S. S. McAllister, "Breast Cancer as a Systematic Disease: A View of Metastasis," *Journal of Internal Medicine* 274.2 (2013): 113-126, http://dx.doi.org/10.1111/joim.12084.

26. Zhen Yang, Anapatricia Garcia, Songli Xu, Doris R. Powell, Paula M. Vertino, Shivendra Singh, and Adam I. Marcus, "*Withania somnifera* Root Extract Inhibits Mammary Cancer Metastasis and Epithelial to Mesenchymal Transition," *PLoS ONE* 8.9 (2013), http://doi.org/10.1371/journal.pone.0075069.

27. "Ashwagandha Extract Increases Testosterone and Strength; Reduces Cortisol," Nutrient Journal, last modified December 23, 2016, http://nutrientjournal.com/ashwagandha-extract-testosterone-strength-increase-reduced-cortisol.

28. Ashwinikumar A. Raut et al., "Exploratory Study to Evaluate Tolerability, Safety, and Activity of Ashwagandha (*Withania somnifera*) in Healthy Volunteers," *Journal of Ayurveda and Integrative Medicine* 3.3 (2012): 111-114, http://doi.org/10.4103/0975-9476.100168.

29. Frank W. Booth, Christian K. Roberts, and Matthew J. Layne, "Lack of Exercise Is a Major Cause of Chronic Illness," *Comprehensive Physiology* 2.2 (2012): 1143-1211, http://doi.org/10.1002/cphy.c110025.

30. A. Paganini-Hill, D. E. Greenia, S. Perry, S. A. Sajjadi, C. H. Kawas, and M. M. Corrada, "Lower Likelihood of Falling at Age 90+ Is Associated with Daily Exercise a Quarter of a Century Earlier: The 90+ Study," *Age and Ageing* 46.6 (2017): 951-957, https://doi.org/10.1093/ageing/afx039.

31. Lynette L. Craft and Frank M. Perna, "The Benefits of Exercise for the Clinically Depressed," *The Primary Care Companion to the Journal of Clinical Psychiatry* 6.3 (2004): 104-111, https://www.ncbi.nlm.nih.gov/pmc/articles/PMC474733/#i1523-5998-6-3-104-b19.

32. Craft and Perna, "The Benefits of Exercise."

33. Larry Husten, "Merck Pleads Guilty and Pays $950 Million for Illegal Promotion of Vioxx," *Forbes*, November 22, 2011, https://www.forbes.com/sites/larryhusten/2011/11/22/merck-pleads-guilty-and-pays-950-million-for-illegal-promotion-of-vioxx.

34. Siri Carpenter, "That Gut Feeling," *American Psychological Association* 43.8 (2012): 50, http://www.apa.org/monitor/2012/09/gut-feeling.aspx.

35. Nora D. Volkow, "America's Addition to Opioids: Heroin and Prescription Drug Abuse," National Institute on Drug Abuse, May 14, 2014, https://www.drugabuse.gov/about-nida/legislative-activities/testimony-to-congress/2016/americas-addiction-to-opioids-heroin-prescription-drug-abuse.

36. M. Warner, L. H. Chen, D. M. Makuc, R. N. Anderson, and A. M. Miniño, "Drug Poisoning Deaths in the United States, 1980-2008," NCHS Data Brief, December 2011, https://www.cdc.gov/nchs/data/databriefs/db81.pdf.

37. Josh Katz, "Drug Deaths in America Are Rising Faster Than Ever," *New York Times*, June 5, 2017, https://www.nytimes.com/interactive/2017/06/05/upshot/opioid-epidemic-drug-overdose-deaths-are-rising-faster-than-ever.html.

38. Richard Pérez-Peña, "Ohio Sues Drug Makers, Saying They Aided Opioid Epidemic," *New York Times*, May 31, 2017, https://www.nytimes.com/2017/05/31/us/ohio-sues-pharmaceutical-drug-opioid-epidemic-mike-dewine.html.

39. Alana Semuels, "Are Pharmaceutical Companies to Blame for the Opioid Epidemic?" *The Atlantic*, June 2, 2017, https://www.theatlantic.com/business/archive/2017/06/lawsuit-pharmaceutical-companies-opioids/529020.

40. T. Conrozier, P. Mathieu, M. Bonjean, J. F. Marc, J. L. Renevier, and J. C. Balblanc, "A Complex of Three Natural Anti-inflammatory Agents Provides Relief of Osteoarthritis Pain," *Alternative Therapies in Health and Medicine* 20.1 (2014): 32-7, https://www.ncbi.nlm.nih.gov/pubmed/24473984.

41. Irving Kirsch, Brett J. Deacon, Tania B. Huedo-Medina, Alan Scoboria, Thomas J. Moore, and Blair T. Johnson, "Initial Severity and Antidepressant Benefits: A Meta-

Analysis of Data Submitted to the Food and Drug Administration," *PLOS Medicine* 5.2 (February 26, 2008): e45, https://doi.org/10.1371/journal.pmed.0050045.

42. M. Maes, I. Mihaylova, M. Kubera, M. Uytterhoeven, N. Vrydags, and E. Bosmans, "Lower Plasma Coenzyme Q10 in Depression: A Marker for Treatment Resistance and Chronic Fatigue in Depression and a Risk Factor to Cardiovascular Disorder in That Illness," *Neuroendocrinology Letters* 30.4 (2009): 462-9, https://www.ncbi.nlm.nih.gov/pubmed/20010493.

43. H. Tiemeier, H. R. van Tuijl, A. Hofman, J. Meijer, A. J. Kiliaan, and M. M. Breteler, "Vitamin B12, Folate, and Homocysteine in Depression: the Rotterdam Study," *American Journal of Psychiatry* 159.12 (2002): 2099-101, https://doi.org/10.1176/appi.ajp.159.12.2099.

44. J. McGrath, K. Saari, H. Hakko et al., "Vitamin D Supplementation during the First Year of Life and Risk of Schizophrenia: A Finnish Birth Cohort Study," *Schizophrenia Research* 67.2-3 (2004): 237-45, http://dx.doi.org/10.1016/j.schres.2003.08.005.

45. Meghan Meehan and Sue Penckofer, "The Role of Vitamin D in the Aging Adult," *Journal of Aging and Gerontology* 2.2 (2014): 60-71, http://doi.org/10.12974/2309-6128.2014.02.02.1.

46. O. Bruni et al., "L-5-Hydroxytryptophan Treatment of Sleep Terrors in Children," *European Journal of Pediatrics* 163.7 (2004): 402-407; J. Pellow et al., "Complementary and Alternative Medical Therapies for Children with Attention-Deficit/Hyperactivity Disorder (ADHD)," *Alternative Medicine Review: A Journal of Clinical Therapeutics* 16.4 (2011): 323-337.

47. K. Linde, M. M. Berner and L. Kriston, "St John's Wort for Major Depression," Cochrane Database of Systematic Reviews 8.4 (2008), https://doi.org/10.1002/14651858.CD000448.pub3.

48. S. B. Sartori, N. Whittle, A. Hetzenauer, and N. Singewald, "Magnesium Deficiency Induces Anxiety and HPA Axis Dysregulation: Modulation by Therapeutic Drug Treatment," *Neuropharmacology* 62.1 (2012): 304-312, http://doi.org/10.1016/j.neuropharm.2011.07.027; Neil Bernard Boyle, Claire Lawton, and Louise Dye, "The Effects of Magnesium Supplementation on Subjective Anxiety and Stress—A Systematic Review," *Nutrients* 9.5 (2017): 429, http://doi.org/10.3390/nu9050429; G. A. Eby and K. L. Eby, "Rapid Recovery from Major Depression Using Magnesium Treatment," *Medical Hypotheses* 67.2 (2006): 362-70, http://dx.doi.org/10.1016/j.mehy.2006.01.047.

49. Stephen Bent, Amy Padula, Dan Moore, Michael Patterson, and Wolf Mehling, "Valerian for Sleep: A Systematic Review and Meta-Analysis," *The American Journal of Medicine* 119.12 (2006): 1005-1012, http://doi.org/10.1016/j.amjmed.2006.02.026.

50. "Valerian," University of Maryland Medical Center, accessed October 25, 2017, http://www.umm.edu/health/medical/altmed/herb/valerian.

51. "Passionflower," University of Maryland Medical Center, accessed October 25, 2017, http://www.umm.edu/health/medical/altmed/herb/passionflower.

52. Fereshteh Mehraein, Maryam Sarbishegi, and Anahita Aslani, "Evaluation of Effect of Oleuropein on Skin Wound Healing in Aged Male Balb/c Mice," *Cell Journal* 16.1 (2014): 25-30, https://www.ncbi.nlm.nih.gov/pmc/articles/PMC3933436.

53. P. Perugini, M. Vettor, C. Rona et al., "Efficacy of Oleuropein against UVB Irradiation: Preliminary Evaluation," *International Journal of Cosmetic Science* 30.2 (2008): 113-120, https://doi.org/10.1111/j.1468-2494.2008.00424.x.

Index